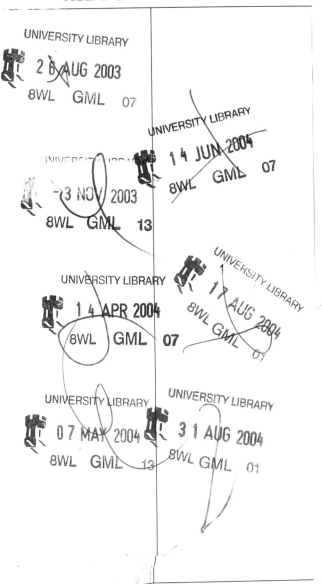
This book may be recalled before the above date.

Finals in Surgery

Commissioning Editor: Laurence Hunter
Project Development Manager: Sarah Keer-Keer
Project Manager: Nancy Arnott
Designer: Erik Bigland
Cartoons: Charles Simpson
Illustrations: Paul Richardson and Charles Simpson

Finals in Surgery

A Guide to Success in Clinical Surgery

Alastair M Thompson
BSc (Hons) MD FRCSEd (Gen)
Senior Lecturer and Honorary Consultant Surgeon,
Department of Surgery, University of Dundee, Dundee

Kenneth G M Park
MD FRCSEd
Consultant Surgeon,
Aberdeen Royal Infirmary, Aberdeen

SECOND EDITION

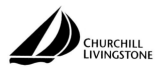
CHURCHILL
LIVINGSTONE

EDINBURGH LONDON NEW YORK PHILADELPHIA ST LOUIS SYDNEY
TORONTO 2001

CHURCHILL LIVINGSTONE
An imprint of Elsevier Science Limited

First published 1997
Second edition 2001
Reprinted 2002

ISBN 0-443-07005-9   *I O O3221555*

British Library Cataloguing in Publication Data
A catalogue record for this book is available from the British Library.

Library of Congress Cataloging in Publication Data
A catalog record for this book is available from the Library of Congress.

Note
Medical knowledge is constantly changing. As information becomes available,
changes in treatment, procedures, equipment and the use of drugs become
necessary. The authors and publisher have, as far as it is possible, taken care to
ensure that the information given in the text is accurate and up-to-date. However,
readers are strongly advised to confirm that the information, especially with
regard to drug usage, complies with current legislation and standards of practice.

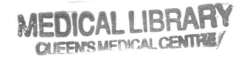
The
publisher's
policy is to use
**paper manufactured
from sustainable forests**

Printed in China

Preface

This book has been written to help you pass your surgical finals. It is not intended as a complete textbook of surgery. However, it should guide you as to what to expect in surgical finals, assist in your revision and suggest ways of answering common questions. While much of the book concentrates on traditional long and short cases, the same approach is very effective in Objective Structured Clinical Examinations (OSCEs). There is a section on topics which may come up in any part of the exam and some examples of radiology designed to complement those in the companion volume *Final MB*.

At the end of many chapters, there are key questions to give you practice with examiner's favourites. These also act as revision questions for the chapter — try them out with your colleagues before the exam.

We hope that you will find this book helps you to prepare for surgical finals and that some of the concepts may be useful in your future clinical practice.

2001

AMT
KGMP

Acknowledgements

The authors wish to thank Dr Laura Wilkinson, Consultant Radiologist, Gartnavel General Hospital, Mr Steve Wigmore, Lecturer in Surgery, University of Edinburgh and Dr Fenton Wallis, Senior Registrar in Radiology, Aberdeen Royal Infirmary, for constructive criticisms and contributions to the text. We also thank the many final year and postgraduate surgical students from Dundee, Edinburgh, Aberdeen, Dublin and Christchurch (New Zealand), who made helpful suggestions in preparing the first edition and who have allowed us to modify and improve the text for this second edition.

Contents

PART 1

GENERAL PRINCIPLES

1

The exam in general

Depending on whether or not you want to be a surgeon, surgery represents either the pinnacle of human achievement or a specialty populated by sociopaths of varying degrees of adaptation. In either case, surgical examinations are a hurdle that must be overcome.

The aims of this book are to describe a simple and logical approach to surgical examinations and to give examples of common topics and questions to help you to overcome this hurdle. Some of the content may also be useful after you have graduated. However, this book is intended not as a textbook of surgery, but as a helping hand during the few weeks before finals.

WHAT IS EXPECTED OF YOU

During clinical examinations. It is important to realize that it is not just factual knowledge that is required. The examiners will be assessing your:

- ability to take a history
- examination technique
- presentation skills
- core knowledge
- deductive reasoning
- communication skills and attitude to patients.

During different sections of your exam more emphasis is placed on certain aspects of surgery; in the clinicals the emphasis is quite rightly on clinical skills. Core knowledge is more appropriately tested in your written papers.

PREPARATION FOR THE EXAM

There may be times when you think that you will never know enough to pass an exam (in whatever subject), but fortunately most students are wrong in this respect! Good preparation can minimize the stress caused by finals. A reasonable amount of effort, inspiring teaching, reliable books, consistent attendance at lectures, seminars and tutorials, and above all exposure to real patients with real problems throughout the undergraduate teaching programme will help you to get through finals.

For textbooks in surgery, small is beautiful, although a text which is too small may not cover the subject adequately for the purpose of passing finals. Select undergraduate textbooks which you find readable; choose a book on clinical examination/surgical signs and find another book aimed at getting you through the exam (if you're reading this, you have made a good choice!).

A good way of learning is to browse through your books, looking up topics you have covered that day on the ward or in teaching sessions. This helps most people to consolidate information, so that key concepts and principles are retained for much longer than when topics or lists are memorized in isolation. Note down any points that you don't really understand and raise them with your fellow students (who are probably puzzled by the same things) and with your teachers on the surgical wards (who may also have to think quite hard). It is better to understand principles on which you can later hang a few facts than to memorize a few facts out of context. This philosophy underlies the increasing emphasis on problem-based learning as opposed to the retention of vast amounts of information, most of which will be forgotten within hours of completing an exam.

During the few days before your exams, ensure that you are familiar with the topics which are usually covered. Being an expert on heart transplantation is of no advantage if you know little about hip fractures, colorectal cancer or thyroid swellings: the former will not come up in finals, the other three topics almost certainly will. If you have a few minutes to spare (unlikely though this may seem), looking through the tables and illustrations in the books you have used is well worthwhile.

Finally, getting a good night's sleep before the exam is more valuable than trying to cram a few extra facts into a tired, caffeine-saturated brain. An alert candidate with a little knowledge is likely to think more clearly, answer questions more lucidly and fare better in the exam than a sleep-deprived swot. Remember the examiners are assessing you and your ability to think logically – this is more likely to impress than one or two extra facts. Sleep deprivation is not a compulsory part of the undergraduate curriculum and is becoming less and less common even for junior hospital doctors.

Failure in surgical finals is guaranteed if you arrive after the exam has finished. Make sure you know where (not just which hospital, but which ward) and when the exam will take place. Set out in good time: it is better to arrive an hour early and approach the exam outwardly composed than to worry that the traffic is making you late and arrive as a ruffled, sweating heap with your mind in a turmoil. If it looks as if you are going to be late, try to phone; if you are late, make apologies: in some situations, the examiners may try to accommodate you.

PERSONAL PRESENTATION

In most clinical exams, including surgical ones, tradition dictates that you dress smartly but comfortably and that you present yourself in a recently-washed state. Dirty fingernails and hands or an untamed head or face of hair are not likely to appeal to either the examiners or the patients. While a tee-shirt and shorts may seem right on a hot day, the jacket and tie or 'sensible' blouse and skirt are more likely to get the examiners and patients looking upon you with confidence as a future doctor. This is not an occasion for experimenting with the latest fad in fashion! Some institutions suggest a white coat as standard attire in the exam, but the above points still apply. Whether you wear normal clothing or a white coat, a clear name-badge can be helpful in identifying yourself to the examiners and patients.

EQUIPMENT

For a surgical exam you do not need to appear laden with heavy-duty medical equipment, prepared for every eventuality. The key essentials for a basic surgical exam are your eyes, ears, hands and brain. To complement these, you need a watch, a stethoscope, a measuring tape, a pen-torch, and a pen and paper. Anything else you need should be provided, including a tendon hammer, a

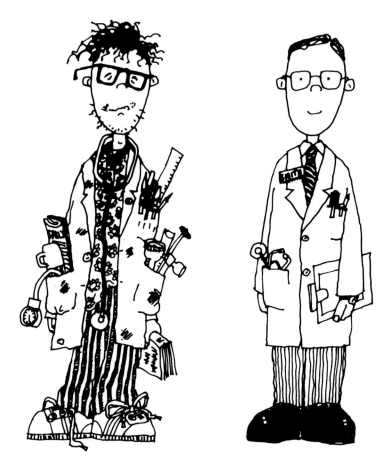

Exam candidates should be presentable and carry only the essentials for surgical finals.

tuning fork, cotton wool, disposable needles, an ophthalmoscope, a blood pressure cuff, urine testing sticks, a tourniquet and gloves.

EXAMINERS

Examiners come in a variety of shapes, sizes and ages and with a range of countenances. They usually hunt in pairs so as to out-number the candidate! One may be an 'internal' examiner, from the institution running the exam, and the other an 'external' exam-iner from St Elsewhere. Although this pairing can make them seem

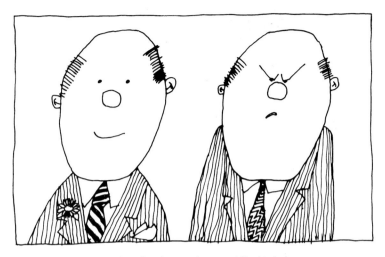

Examiners usually hunt in pairs: the good guy and the bad guy.

pretty intimidating, it is really to ensure fair play. Examiners should introduce themselves to you, and may already know something about the patients you see. If one examiner knows you (from your time on the wards or because you beat him or her in the annual medical school golf competition), he or she may opt to swap places with a colleague or simply to listen. Unfortunately, even if you are to be assessed by an examiner whom you feel may not ensure fair play, it may not be possible to swap with another candidate: check with the person running the exam.

The examiners should mark you according to a schedule, which may be divided into categories such as: approach to the patient; history-taking; clinical examination of the patient; presentational skills; and ability to interpret findings and answer questions.

The examiners will confer with each other after you have left, and will decide what mark to award you for that component of the exam. The various marks you receive will be collated, and borderline candidates (for distinction or pass/fail) may undergo further assessment.

Key points

- Prepare for the exam in good time
- Try to grasp the concepts and principles onto which you can hang facts

- Use books to consolidate information on patients you have seen or topics you have discussed
- Approach the exam rested, smartly dressed and outwardly cool, calm and collected
- Take to the exam a watch, stethoscope, tape, torch, pen and paper
- Remember examiners generally want you to get through the exam

2

The exam in detail

Most patients involved in the clinical exams are either patients in the wards at the time of the exam (preoperative patients, patients admitted for investigation or, occasionally, postoperative patients) or outpatients who have been brought to the hospital to help with the exam (often having a hernia, varicose veins, orthopaedic problems or a skin lesion).

EXAMINATION OF THE PATIENT

Before examining a patient, it is wise to formally introduce yourself (you may have been told the patient's name, but they probably do not know yours), and to establish contact with the patient by shaking hands. This usually gets the patient on your side and shows that you too are human (if a little frightened), and so gets the examination off to a good start. Beware the rare patient who has a painful hand (perhaps with a drip in place) or who has a paralysed right upper limb, an amputation or a congenital limb deformity: you may find yourself shaking their left, instead of their right, hand!

It is traditional to stand at the patient's right-hand side, particularly if you are going to examine the chest or abdomen. This has the advantage of familiarity: if you always approach and examine the patient in the same way, you will have developed a sense of security prior to your exam. Also, you are much more likely to detect abnormalities.

Remember to look for clues, particularly in the traditional long case, during which you are likely to be left with the patient for between 20 minutes and an hour. TPR (temperature/pulse/blood pressure/respiratory rate) charts may show pyrexia or a change in pulse or blood pressure over time. Drug charts may hint at not only the disease(s) the patient has but also their investigation and management. Radiographs are sometimes left with the patient and can give helpful hints as to how the patient has been investigated (look at the envelope containing the radiographs) and even indicate the diagnosis. Some patients have been involved in surgical finals before, and if you strike it lucky with a cooperative patient who knows a lot about his or her condition, the exam can become almost enjoyable. Even so, don't forget to cover the basics.

For both undergraduate and postgraduate clinical examinations, four formats may be used: the long case, short cases, orals and Objective Structured Clinical Examinations (OSCEs). Ensure that you are familiar with the structure of the examinations you are about to sit.

LONG CASE

The traditional surgical long case usually involves the candidate being allocated a patient. You are required to take a history and examine the patient and then present the case, suggest how to investigate the patient and discuss their surgical and non-surgical management. In the long case you will be assessed initially on your presentation skills; thereafter on your ability to think logically about possible diagnoses, appropriate investigations and management.

The secret to performing well in a long case is to take an accurate history with sufficient relevant details and to examine the patient appropriately, paying particular attention to the condition(s) from which the patient suffers. Make short notes as you go, but don't waste time scripting a beautifully written history: the emphasis of the exam is on oral communication of your history-taking and on your clinical examination skills. Having noted the main findings of the history and examination, write down the investigations you would order, then list the treatment options. Beware: patients selected for long cases often suffer from more than one condition (e.g. breast cancer, ischaemic heart disease and osteoarthritis), so you have to remember to outline the relevant findings, investigations and treatments for each condition and indicate how they are interrelated.

Try to set aside 5 minutes before the examiners pounce, so that you can organize your thoughts and present them coherently.

The following is a general scheme for a long case, which you should adapt to suit yourself and should practise many times prior to the exam:

1. history
2. clinical examination
3. summary of patient
4. differential diagnosis
5. investigations
6. management.

History

Write down key words and phrases as you go:

- name and age of patient
- problem(s)/presenting symptom(s)
- systematic enquiry for each problematic system
- past medical/surgical history
- drug history/allergies/alcohol/smoking
- social history, including home circumstances and support
- occupation
- family history
- systematic enquiry for systems not already covered.

Unfortunately not all patients are cooperative: sometimes communication is difficult (e.g. the deaf patient who has lost his teeth, is very talkative, and speaks with a curious accent you can't quite understand); or the patient doesn't really want to participate in the exam (just like you) and takes it out on you. Occasionally, a patient may become unwell during the long case: you should alert the exam supervisor. Nursing staff can be particularly helpful, especially in an emergency. The patient may, however, understand the exam situation and spill the beans freely to you (including all the investigations and treatments to date if you're lucky). Even so, ensure that you have asked all the relevant questions: it is all too easy to accept at face value all that is volunteered and miss out on some essential points. For example, a patient who tells you his gallstones were revealed by ultrasound scanning and that he has had pancreatitis still needs to be asked about alcohol consumption.

There are patients with complex histories who may happily fill an hour by just giving you their life story. With practice (so do not attempt it for the first time in the exam) it is possible to obtain part

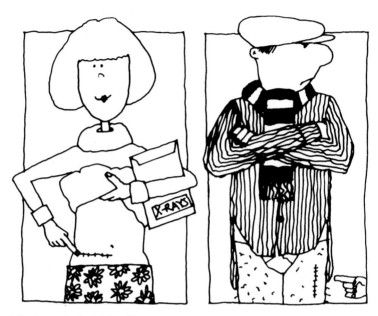

Patients can be helpful or, like you, may not really want to participate in the exam

of the patient's history while you perform the physical examination: you may see this being done in outpatient clinics or on ward rounds.

Clinical examination

Note abnormal findings (see Fig. 2.1):

- general features (jaundice, anaemia, cyanosis, clubbing, oedema, lymphadenopathy, cachexia, etc.)
- head and neck examination
- cardiovascular system
- respiratory system
- breast examination
- abdominal examination (no rectal examination in the exam)
- limb and back examination
- neurological examination (central and peripheral).

One way to approach the examination in a long case is illustrated in Figure 2.1. As you proceed through the patient's examination, note down positive and important findings.

1. **Gross cognitive assessment**
   • ? orientated
2. **Gross physical assessment**
   • ? cachexia
   • obesity
   • mobility during examination

   6. **Facies**
      • in general
      • jaundice

5. **BP**

4. **Pulse**

3. **Hands**
   • establish contact
   • fingers/nails
   • muscles
   • colour

12. **Abdomen**
    • inspection
      – scars
      – movement
    • palpation
      – tenderness
      – masses
      – organs
      – (rectal examination)
    • percussion
    • auscultation

16. **Urinalysis**
    Temperature

17. **Check** that you
    • have the positive findings in note form
    • can present the case in a coherent manner

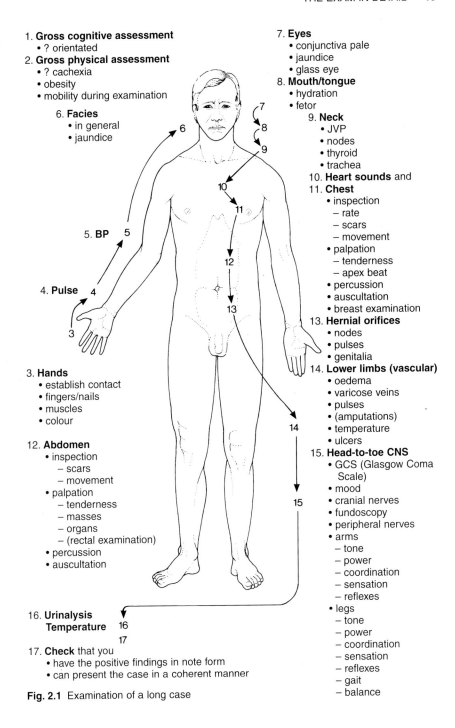

7. **Eyes**
   • conjunctiva pale
   • jaundice
   • glass eye
8. **Mouth/tongue**
   • hydration
   • fetor
9. **Neck**
   • JVP
   • nodes
   • thyroid
   • trachea
10. **Heart sounds** and
11. **Chest**
    • inspection
      – rate
      – scars
      – movement
    • palpation
      – tenderness
      – apex beat
    • percussion
    • auscultation
    • breast examination
13. **Hernial orifices**
    • nodes
    • pulses
    • genitalia
14. **Lower limbs (vascular)**
    • oedema
    • varicose veins
    • pulses
    • (amputations)
    • temperature
    • ulcers
15. **Head-to-toe CNS**
    • GCS (Glasgow Coma Scale)
    • mood
    • cranial nerves
    • fundoscopy
    • peripheral nerves
    • arms
      – tone
      – power
      – coordination
      – sensation
      – reflexes
    • legs
      – tone
      – power
      – coordination
      – sensation
      – reflexes
      – gait
      – balance

Fig. 2.1 Examination of a long case

Summary of patient

- Introduction (e.g. 'Mr John Knox, a 72-year-old former preacher . . .')
- Problems (e.g. '. . . who presents with . . . (one sentence)')
- Main findings ('On examination . . . (one or two sentences)').

Differential diagnosis

- Principal problem(s)
- Other problem(s).

Investigations

The emphasis, when discussing investigations, must be on:

1. Starting with the simple, non-invasive tests – building on these accordingly
2. Investigations appropriate to the patient's condition.

Choose from the following list the appropriate tests for the patient you have seen:

Urine dipstick test
- biochemistry/microbiology
- pregnancy test

Faeces
- occult blood
- microbiology
- tests of gastrointestinal function

Blood tests, including:
- haematology, coagulation
- biochemistry
- microbiology
- immunology
- blood transfusion
- hormone levels

Cardiology
- ECG
- echocardiography

Radiology
- skull and cervical spine radiograph
- chest radiograph
- abdominal/pelvic radiograph

- limb radiograph
- contrast studies of:
  - gastrointestinal tract
  - vascular tree
  - urological system
- ultrasound and Doppler scanning
- computed tomography
- magnetic resonance imaging
- radionuclide imaging

Surgical studies
- upper endoscopy
- endoscopic retrograde cholangiopancreatography (ERCP)
- proctoscopy
- rigid sigmoidoscopy
- flexible sigmoidoscopy/colonoscopy

Physiological studies
- upper gastrointestinal tract
- lower gastrointestinal tract
- urinary system
- nervous system

Pathology
- cytology
- biopsy.

For example, a patient with jaundice should have urinalysis, faecal occult blood testing, haematology, coagulation, biochemistry followed by ultrasound before proceeding to ERCP.

Management

- Conservative measures (modify diet, stop smoking, etc.)
- Medical therapy (fluids, analgesia, etc.)
- Chemotherapy
- Radiotherapy
- Surgery.

Approach to a long case

For a long case, allow yourself approximately the times shown in Table 2.1.

Obviously, there is a lot of similarity between approaching a long case in surgical and medical exams. Some medical schools combine

Table 2.1 Use of time in a long case		
Length of case	1 hour	30 min
History	20 min	10 min
Examination	20 min	10 min
Summary/differential diagnosis	5 min	3 min
Investigations/plan management	5 min	3 min
Organize/go over presentation/think through some questions	10 min	4 min

the two and give you a single long case, usually cunningly selecting a patient with both medical and surgical problems.

Practise seeing patients under simulated exam conditions in the lead up to your exam, recording the information listed above and then presenting the patient to a fellow student or qualified doctor. A competently conducted history and examination, thoughtfully presented to your examiners, will give you the best possible basis on which to succeed in finals.

Presentation

The oral presentation about the patient you have just seen is something that becomes easier with practice. Aim to present the exam patient in the way you have previously presented patients to your fellow students and teachers. Speak slowly and clearly, and use medical terminology precisely, so that the examiners can follow you. Emphasize the positive points and if there are a number of problems or disease processes, deal with these one at a time. Avoid reeling off a list of negative findings: carefully chosen phrases like 'on systematic enquiry, there were no abnormal genitourinary or neurological symptoms' or 'on examination, the cardiovascular and respiratory systems were otherwise normal' can be used to good effect.

Don't be put off by apparent inattention on the part of your examiners: they may still be listening carefully. Examiners can be quite irritating and may interrupt your masterful presentation to ask further questions. They may simply want to clarify a point. Alternatively, they may launch into questioning because it has become clear to them that you have no idea about the patient (unlikely), or because you have convinced them that your history/ examination technique is adequate and they can't wait to start quizzing your finely tuned, razor-sharp mind! Occasionally, you may have identified things in the history or examination that the examiners hadn't spotted or you may have missed an important feature: the examiners will then feel entitled to take you back to review the patient. Even if you have got something wrong, the situation may be retrieved by staying outwardly calm, doing as the examiners ask, admitting your mistake and changing your answer if necessary.

SHORT CASE

In many ways, short cases are a rehearsal for your professional life as a hospital doctor in Outpatient or Accident and Emergency Departments, or for general practice surgeries. One excellent way to prepare for short cases is to attend surgical outpatient clinics. This will give you practice, sometimes under the eyes of your future examiners, at taking a concise history (with perhaps three key open-ended questions); at examining the relevant systems, speedily but accurately; and at establishing the symptoms, signs and underlying condition(s). The emphasis in short cases is on how you interrogate a patient, given a starting point, or how you examine a system. The more you have practised examining and are familiar with a system of examination, the more relaxed you will seem and the better you will perform. You will then come to your finals in the knowledge that you can confidently and competently address most of the short case topics likely to come up in the exam.

As mentioned already, it is worthwhile introducing yourself to the patient and establishing contact by shaking hands. In the few seconds that this takes, you may get some clues about the condition(s) from which the patient suffers – for example, a walking stick or obvious musculoskeletal deformities may suggest that the patient has had orthopaedic treatment for arthritis.

You may be asked to take a brief history (e.g. by asking 'What are the main problems that have brought you to the hospital?') or simply to examine the patient. Listen carefully to what your examiner asks.

Clinical examination

Examination should follow the scheme:

- exposure/position
- inspection
- palpation
- percussion
- auscultation.

This is modified for orthopaedic examinations to:

- exposure/position
- look
- feel
- move.

Exposure/position means that you need to ensure that clothing has been removed from the part of the body you are about to inspect. Both limbs should be exposed in the case of a limb problem (without socks remaining to hide something relevant); the abdomen should be exposed from nipple to groin; and for the examination of the head and neck, the shirt should be removed, and not just the collar loosened, to allow adequate visualization of the neck. The patient should be positioned so that you can examine the appropriate area and he or she is comfortable (and hence remains cooperative).

Before palpation, always ask if there is any tenderness. Apparently comfortable patients can turn you into a nervous wreck if you grasp a tender, rheumatoid limb.

Approach to a short case

Pay attention to what the examiner actually asks you: compare 'Describe this skin lesion' (a specific question) with 'Examine this patient's groin': in the latter, there may be any number of problems, and you need to go through the examination scheme for the groin carefully. To ensure that the examiners appreciate what you are demonstrating, you may wish to talk your way through a short case. An examiner may interrupt your examination and ask you about your findings so far and how you would proceed. Alternatively, an examiner may direct you to repeat or perform a particular manoeuvre to get you to elicit a specific sign.

While you examine a patient, be alert for clues which may suggest the diagnosis (e.g. a glass of water to assist swallowing during examination of the thyroid). It is worthwhile trying to think through some of the things you may be asked about. For example, a palpable thyroid lump may prompt you to think of the symptoms and signs of hyperthyroidism, or finger clubbing may alert you to recall the various possible causes of clubbing. This will give you the edge when the examiner asks those same questions!

ORAL EXAMS

Most examiners will ask questions (and expect answers!) stemming from your presentation of the long case or as part of the short cases but in some medical schools there are separate face-to-face question and answer sessions, usually lasting 5–20 minutes. Sometimes, the oral exam can cover anaesthetics, microbiology relevant to surgery, laboratory investigations (biochemistry, haematology) or pathology.

As for the clinical exam, an appropriate standard of dress and degree of decorum are required for oral (viva voce) exams. Before, during and after this part of an exam, you may feel nervous, frightened, intimidated, and completely ignorant of all things surgical, and wish that a hole in the ground would swallow you up. This is very common! Most examiners understand this, and should put you at your ease by starting off with a simple question.

The golden rules for oral examinations are to: wait for the examiner to finish asking the question; think briefly before you open your mouth; and then speak clearly. Start with general features and then go on to specific points, and mention common conditions before rarities. Giving scorpion stings as a cause of pancreatitis suggests you are clueless about its common causes (alcohol and gallstones), not that you are well read. If you know a lot about the topic you have been asked about, keep talking – the examiner will interrupt you soon enough.

When asked about the management of a particular condition, it is worthwhile starting with 'Having taken a history and examined the patient . . .'. If asked about the treatment of a patient, start with 'Having taken a history, examined and appropriately investigated this man with colonic carcinoma . . .'.

If an examiner challenges something you have said, either stick to your statement ('Yes, femoral hernias are more common in women than in men') or correct the error you may have made

('I should have said femoral hernias are more common in women than in men, not the other way round'). Sometimes examiners may say you are wrong: it is better to accept their judgement (whatever you may secretly think!) and move on to the next topic than to enter into an argument which you cannot win, even if you are right. In effect, the examiners make the rules, field the opposing team and act as referee. If the questions get difficult, this usually means that you are doing well, so don't be discouraged. The examiners may even start to impart some of their own wisdom to you!

When answering the questions, try to structure your answers as follows:

- history (symptoms)
- examination (signs, including urinalysis)
- investigations (blood, radiology, microbiology, pathology, special tests such as endoscopy)
- diagnosis
- management/treatment (conservative, medical, chemotherapy, radiotherapy or surgical).

Even if you know little about the topic in question, by answering in this structured way you may be able to scrape together enough information to satisfy the examiners. The sequence of history (symptoms), examination (signs), investigations, diagnosis and management/treatment forms the basic structure for not only examinations but also medical practice in real life in outpatient clinics, emergency rooms and general practice surgeries. So this simple approach to clinical problems (not just in surgery) can help to get you through life as a medical graduate as well as through exams.

OBJECTIVE STRUCTURED CLINICAL EXAMINATIONS (OSCEs)

An Objective Structured Clinical Examination (OSCE) is, as the name suggests, designed to assess individual students objectively with structured questions. By using a predetermined, structured marking regime and patients (or actors) who have known clinical histories and examination findings, the OSCE should standardize what students are asked and the way they are marked, cutting out the subjective and variable standards of conventional exams. An OSCE exam may comprise several different topics with the candidates moving between individual stations. For example, there may be ten stations, two on history taking (jaundiced patient, change in bowel habit), three on clinical examination (chest, lower limb, abdomen), three on investigations (an abdominal film, some blood results, urine test), one on communication skills and one on cardiopulmonary resuscitation. Thus an OSCE-style examination may test many of the skills and techniques outlined earlier in this chapter which you would apply to traditional long case/short case/oral examinations.

In the OSCE you may be asked to take a relevant history, with the examiner marking your questions relating to the history and/or investigations and treatment of the patient's condition. You are thus being tested on how good your history taking skills are against the same marking schedule which will be used for the other candidates. Alternatively, you may be asked to 'examine the abdomen of this man who presented with . . .'. Marks are allocated for elements of the examination technique correctly performed, positive clinical findings noted, and answers to questions about investigations and treatment. Similarly you may be asked to inspect a limb for signs of acute ischaemia. As you state the features that you find, the examiner will award the marks indicated on the marking schedule for pale (1); pulseless (1); painful (1); paraesthesia (1) and perishingly cold (1), the maximum score being 5 marks. There may be questions on the causes of the ischaemia, complications and/or the possible treatments: conservative measures (stop smoking, increase exercise) (2); medical therapy (1); surgical therapy (angioplasty, arterial reconstruction, amputation) (3).

There should, theoretically, be no subjective component of the marking schedule – eliminating the variations in the questions the examiners ask and the level of knowledge they expect, and thereby making it a fairer exam. However, time constraints and examiner boredom limit the use of OSCEs in some medical schools.

Key points

- Practice is the best way to success in clinical examination
- Always introduce yourself to the patient
- Look for clues (e.g. walking stick, charts, radiographs, glass of water)
- Speak slowly and clearly, and use precise medical terminology

- **Long case**: allocate appropriate lengths of time to:
  - history
  - examination
  - summary/differential diagnosis
  - investigations/plan of management
  - organize/go over presentation/think through some questions
- **Short case**: remember:
  - exposure/position
  - inspection
  - palpation
  - percussion
  - auscultation
- **Short case/oral/OSCE**:
  - listen to the question
  - think
  - answer the question posed

3

The surgical sieve

The overall scheme for the assessment and management of any patient can be summarized as follows:

- history (symptoms)
- examination (signs, including urinalysis)
- investigations (blood, radiology, microbiology, pathology, special tests such as endoscopy)
- diagnosis
- management.

Once you have an idea of the patient's problem(s), it is possible to use the 'surgical sieve' to work out the underlying pathological processes, likely diagnoses and possible management.

The traditional long case is most likely to test your ability to put all of these steps together, however short cases and OSCEs may test aspects of this. For example, given that this patient fell on her outstretched arm, can you comment on her X-Ray? What is the diagnosis? What are the management options?

CLASSIFICATION OF PROBLEMS

In the case of each problem that you have identified in the history or on examination, consider whether the condition is congenital or acquired and which system(s) it has affected.

Conditions

Congenital

- Inherited
- Developmental

Acquired

- Infective
  - acute/chronic
  - bacterial/viral/other
- Neoplastic
  - benign/malignant
  - primary/secondary
- Inflammatory
  - acute/chronic
  - local/generalized
  - granulomatous/non-granulomatous
- Traumatic
  - acute/chronic
- Vascular
  - acute/chronic
  - peripheral/central
  - arterial/venous
- Endocrine
  - by gland/by mechanism
  - underactive/overactive
- Metabolic
  - acute/chronic
- Autoimmune
  - local/generalized
- Degenerative
- Miscellaneous

Systems

- Cardiovascular
- Respiratory
- Gastrointestinal
- Genitourinary
- Central nervous system
- Peripheral nervous system
- Locomotor
- Endocrine
- Skin

For example, in the case of a patient who presents with a breast lump, the lump may be infective, neoplastic, inflammatory, or traumatic and is affecting an endocrine responsive organ. When listing your differential diagnosis, start with the most common cause and work your way down to less common causes.

Another way of classifying conditions, particularly applicable to the mechanical obstruction of a tubular organ (such as the gastrointestinal tract), is based on whether the pathology causing symptoms lies:

- within the lumen
- within the wall
- outside the wall.

For example, a patient with dysphagia due to obstruction of the oesophagus may have: a bolus obstruction due to a food bolus lodging in the lumen of the oesophagus, or a malignant stricture in the wall of the oesophagus, or else external compression from a primary lung tumour.

MANAGEMENT

Having worked out the possible diagnoses, a systematic approach should be used to consider the treatment options for each condition in a particular patient. Try applying this scheme to patients you meet on the wards:

- conservative treatment
  - prophylactic (e.g. take exercise)
  - stop (e.g. smoking)
  - start (e.g. high fibre diet)
- medical treatment
  - prophylactic (e.g. immunization)
  - curative (e.g. antibiotics)
  - maintenance of function (e.g. digoxin)
- chemotherapy
  - adjuvant (e.g. breast or colon cancer)
  - curative (e.g. teratoma)
  - palliative (e.g. liver metastases)
- radiotherapy
  - adjuvant (e.g. breast cancer)
  - curative (e.g. basal cell carcinoma)
  - palliative (e.g. bone metastases)
- surgery
  - minimally invasive (e.g. endoscopy, interventional radiology)
  - relieving (e.g. abscess)
  - resectional (e.g. appendix, tumour)
  - reconstructive (e.g. arterial graft).

As an example of the use of this systematic approach, consider the case of a patient with splenomegaly and hypersplenism, secondary to idiopathic thrombocytopenic purpura. Conservative measures alone are unlikely to be of benefit, and neither chemotherapy nor radiotherapy is indicated. Medical options include the use of steroids, and surgical removal of the spleen (by laparoscopy or by open surgery) is also possible.

COMPLICATIONS

Problems related to surgery and its complications can, as well as being classified by condition and system as above, be classed as one or more of:

- preoperative
- intraoperative
- postoperative.

To complicate matters further, any such complications may:

- be localized or systemic
- be a possible consequence of any operation or be specific to a particular operation
- occur in the short term or the long term after the surgery.

For example, a patient with a fractured neck of the femur may have cardiorespiratory disease and may arrive at hospital with hypothermia (preoperative, systemic problems which could exist prior to any operation). Following the intraoperative complication of blood loss (localized problem with systemic effects), postoperatively the patient may develop deep venous thrombosis complicated by pulmonary embolism (localized then systemic problem which may occur after any operation but is more common after hip surgery than after most procedures). Wound infection of the hemiarthroplasty could occur 1 year later (long-term problem specific to joint replacement surgery).

EXAMINERS' FAVOURITES

There are some problems and types of patient which seem to come up time and time again in surgical finals. The top 20 short cases (not in order of importance) probably include:

abdominal mass
basal cell carcinoma
breast lump
bunion
ingrown toenail
jaundice
lipoma
neck lump
palpable liver
peripheral vascular disease

carpal tunnel syndrome
Dupuytren's contracture
ganglion
hernia
pigmented skin lesion
scrotal swelling
sebaceous cyst
stoma
thyroid swelling
varicose veins.

The top five long cases are probably:

abdominal mass
breast cancer
gallstone disease
orthopaedic problem
peripheral vascular disease.

Key points

- **Assessment and management of any patient:**
  - history (symptoms)
  - examination (signs)
  - investigations
  - diagnosis
  - management
- **The surgical sieve** identifies conditions as congenital or acquired, in the case of each organ or system affected
- **Management may be categorized as:**
  - conservative
  - medical
  - chemotherapy
  - radiotherapy
  - surgery
- **Complications** may be grouped as:
  - preoperative/intraoperative/postoperative
  - localized/systemic
  - short-term/long-term

PART 2

APPROACH TO CASES

NB Please note the following symbols which are used throughout this part of the book:

* Indicates cases that frequently crop up in surgical examinations
† indicates cases that are less common
§ indicates more complicated cases that occur only rarely
* Concentrate your efforts on knowing about the common conditions.

4

Skin, lumps and bumps

Skin lesions, lumps and bumps are very common in short cases in surgical finals. This is in part because such problems are common and can be examined repeatedly by different candidates without upsetting the patient, but also because they test things you will have seen before and can be used as a talking point for differential diagnoses and treatment. The best way to prepare for skin lesions, lumps and bumps in the exam is to see and examine many such lesions during your time as an undergraduate. However, this is rarely possible and a good second-best alternative is to look up the appearance and features of the common lesions in one of the many good colour atlases of surgery.

Since these lesions can be present on almost any part of the body, there is some overlap between the topics covered in this chapter and those in Chapters 5, 7 and 9.

HISTORY

You may not get much chance to take a history from a patient with a skin lesion or lump if the examiners are using the case to carry out a spot check on your observational skills. However, the approximate age of the patient and the location of the lesion will be apparent. If you do get the opportunity to ask anything, key questions should cover:

- the duration of the lesion (when it first appeared, whether it has changed since the patient first noticed it)
- any predisposing events (e.g. sun exposure, trauma, insect bite)
- whether the lesion is tender
- whether there has been any change in size, shape or colour (these three points are particularly important if you suspect a melanoma).

Also, ask about:

- any other lesions
- any associated features (e.g. pain in an inflammatory lymph node; intermittent discharge from a sebaceous cyst; pain of cutaneous nerve distribution)
- what treatment has been suggested or administered.

EXAMINATION

Exposure/position

The examination of a lump or skin lesion, like any other clinical examination, needs adequate exposure of not just the lesion but the whole region and the regional lymph nodes before progressing to inspection, palpation, percussion and auscultation.

Inspection

During your general approach and introduction to the patient, you should note any general features of disease (jaundice, cachexia, etc.) that you may comment on later. Look at and describe to the examiner the following features of the lesion(s):

- number (single/multiple)
- position
- size (in cm: use your measuring tape)
- shape
- colour
- outline of the margin
- contour of the surface.

If the skin overlying the lesion appears to be intact, observe whether the skin:

- appears tight (thin, shiny)
- appears discoloured (e.g. bluish, erythematous)
- has obvious associated blood vessels.

In the case of an ulcerated lesion, include comments about:

- the edge (e.g. sloping, punched out, everted, rolled, undermined)
- the base (e.g. whether there is clean granulation tissue or slough. Can you see bone or a tendon?)

- the approximate depth of the ulcer
- the presence or absence of a discharge from the ulcer.

For skin lesions on the limbs, make it obvious to the examiner that you are examining the whole surface of a limb. Ask the patient whether the limb is painful and examine between the toes. Lift up the lower limb to scrutinize its complete circumference, including the heel, and look for other lesions of the skin.

Palpation

Before touching the patient, check whether there is any pain or tenderness.

Feel for a temperature difference between the lesion and the surrounding tissues, traditionally using the back of your fingers. Palpate the lesion very gently to detect any tenderness (tender lumps are unlikely to be in the exam for obvious reasons, but towards the end of an exam, a lump may become tender following examination by several candidates).

Consider the composition of a lump and try to identify whether it is solid or filled with fluid or gas:

- Does it feel hard or soft?
- Is it fluctuant? (The test for fluctuance uses three fingers on a lump which must be at least 2cm in size)
- Can the lump be transilluminated? (Use a pen-torch pressed against the skin)
- Could the lump be vascular?
- Look for pulsatility (which may simply be transmitted)
- Feel whether the lump is expansile
- Feel for a bruit
- Assess whether the lesion can be compressed and whether it refills when released (as does a sapheno varix).

The relationship of a skin lesion or subcutaneous lump to the overlying and surrounding tissues may be the key feature in defining the diagnosis. Decide whether a lesion is in the skin itself or in the subcutaneous tissues, and whether a lump is tethered or even fixed to the deeper structures. An assessment can be made of the fixity of the lump to muscles and fascia by asking the patient to contract the underlying muscles. This can also be useful in assessing whether a lump is mobile in all directions or whether mobility is restricted to one direction. Rarely, a lump may result in pain corresponding to the distribution of a local nerve, or even a distal neurological deficit.

Palpation of the regional lymph nodes should not be forgotten: ask the examiner, and then the patient, for permission to examine the regional lymph nodes. For lesions of the lower limb, buttock and perineum, include the inguinal lymph nodes. For lesions of the upper limb, include the epitrochlear, axillary, infraclavicular and supraclavicular nodes. For lesions of the torso, include the groin, axillary, infraclavicular, supraclavicular and cervical nodes, depending on the site of the lesion. For head and neck lesions, remember to examine not just the lymph node most likely to be involved in drainage, but also the other cervical nodes.

Percussion

Percussion may be useful for detecting resonance, if you suspect that there is a gas-filled viscus within a large lump (for example, a bowel-containing hernia).

Auscultation

Auscultation for a bruit (in the case of a vascular lesion) or bowel sounds should be mentioned to the examiner, and performed, where appropriate.

Further examination

After you have examined a skin lesion or lump you may be asked whether there are any other things you would like to do. This usually either means that you have not examined the lesion adequately or is a hint not to forget the regional lymph nodes. If you suspect that the lesion is part of a systemic disease process (such as metastatic malignancy, lymphoma or sarcoidosis), you should suggest that it would be useful to examine for lymphadenopathy elsewhere or to examine organs (e.g. the breast) for the site of a primary tumour or secondary spread (e.g. to the liver).

Summary

Remember the features of a lump that you should comment upon:

• size
• shape

- colour
- position
- consistency
- fixation to skin and/or deeper structures
- associated features (including regional lymph nodes)

TYPICAL CASES

Some of the lesions you may see are illustrated in Figure 4.1.

Sebaceous cyst*

Key points

- Punctum
- Arises within the skin

The history is usually of a long-standing lump, and may involve intermittent swelling resulting in a cheesy discharge. On examination, a punctum (the opening of the cyst onto the skin surface) is usually visible. The skin is usually immovable over the cyst and tightly adherent to it, because a sebaceous cyst lies within the skin itself.

Sebaceous cysts are frequently found in the scalp, neck, axilla or groin and may be multiple.

A sebaceous cyst is a popular choice for exams, as it needs to be distinguished from a lipoma.

Lipoma*

Key points

- Overlying skin mobile
- Seems fluctuant

A lipoma may be solitary, with a long history of slow growth (sometimes to many cm in size) or there may be multiple lipomata (often 2–4 cm in size). Rarely, lipomata may be tender or may compress surrounding structures. A lipoma may appear to be fluctuant

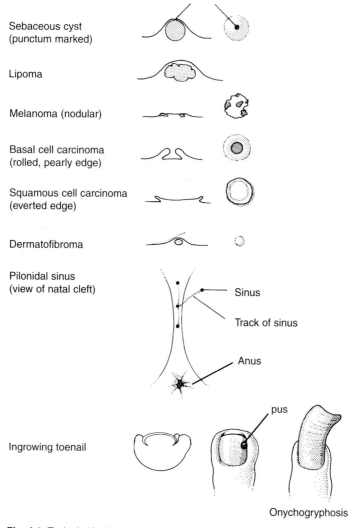

Sebaceous cyst
(punctum marked)

Lipoma

Melanoma (nodular)

Basal cell carcinoma
(rolled, pearly edge)

Squamous cell carcinoma
(everted edge)

Dermatofibroma

Pilonidal sinus
(view of natal cleft)

Sinus

Track of sinus

Anus

pus

Ingrowing toenail

Onychogryphosis

Fig. 4.1 Typical skin lesions

because of the semifluid nature of fat at body temperature. It is often lobulated in outline. It lies in the subcutaneous tissues, and sometimes passes down through a fascial plane, which results in tethering to the underlying tissues. The skin over a lipoma should be freely mobile and this feature, together with the absence of a punctum, distinguishes it from a sebaceous cyst. A lipoma may recur after resection, and so you may see a scar related to the lump.

Lymph node*

Key points

- Regional or generalized lymphadenopathy
- Consider the region that the nodes drain

Single or multiple lymph nodes, in one or several groups, are common short cases because of the frequency of lymphadenopathy in clinical practice. The most important features of lymphadenopathy are the position, number, size, consistency and distribution of the lymph nodes. As a rough guide, soft lymph nodes are probably benign; a rubbery consistency suggests lymphoma; and hard lumps suggest metastatic carcinoma. Wherever the nodes are sited, it is imperative that you ask the examiner whether you can examine the region which the nodes drain: axillary nodes drain the upper limb, breasts and torso; cervical nodes drain inside the mouth as well as the head and neck; and groin nodes drain the lower limb and perineum. Ask whether you can examine other node groups, and enquire about systemic symptoms.

Lymphadenopathy in the context of typical surgical cases is discussed in Chapters 5, 7 and 9.

Differentiation between sebaceous cyst, lipoma and lymph node*

It is an exam favourite to test that you can differentiate between a sebaceous cyst, a lipoma and a lymph node. This may not be as easy as it sounds, but some helpful hints are given in Table 4.1.

Table 4.1   Features of common lumps

Lesion	Sebaceous cyst	Lipoma	Lymph node
Size	5 mm–2 cm	1–10+ cm	5 mm–2+ cm
Shape	Spherical	Disc	Bean-like
Colour	Skin may be red	Normal skin	Normal skin
Consistency	Soft or hard	Soft/fluctuant	Firm or hard
Position	Scalp/axilla/neck	Trunk/limbs	Neck/axilla/groin
Fixation	To skin	?To muscle	?To muscle
Associated features	Punctum		Likely to be
	Cheesy exudate		multiple

Ganglion*

Key points

• Associated with tendon sheath or joint

A ganglion (a gelatinous fluid collection related to a tendon sheath or joint) is an exam favourite and makes a good case for 'on the spot' diagnosis. Ganglia are usually single lumps, 1–4 cm in size. They are either soft and fluctuant or quite hard and tense, with a smooth, often rounded, outline. Ganglia are associated with a tendon sheath or joint, and are usually located around the wrist, on the dorsum of the hand or over the dorsum of the ankle. The overlying skin is usually mobile, and it may be possible to transilluminate a large ganglion.

Treatment used to be to strike the ganglion with a Bible (or other heavy object); alternatively the ganglion can be burst by injection of local anaesthetic and steroid. However, if it recurs or if the patient wishes to have the ganglion removed, surgical excision is now recommended. Ganglia are prone to recur if incompletely excised, so look for an adjacent scar.

Melanoma*

Key points

• Changes in size, shape, colour
• Examine regional nodes

A pigmented skin lesion should be thought of as a melanoma in an exam, although it may well be simply a naevus (intradermal, or more rarely, junctional, compound or juvenile). Changes in size, shape or colour are the most frequently observed features of a pigmented lesion which turns out to be a melanoma. Itching, bleeding and a history of exposure to sunshine may also be noted.

Any of the following types of melanoma may turn up in the final exam: lentigo maligna melanoma (a large flat lesion, usually on an elderly person's face, which may show areas of differing pigmentation also known as Hutchinson's Melanotic freckle); superficial spreading melanoma (irregular border, areas of differing pigmentation, acral lentiginous melanoma (on the soles or palms); or nodular melanoma. Remember that all of these lesions may occur at any age (with the exception of lentigo maligna melanoma which occurs age ≥ 40 years).

You should examine the lesion and describe:

- its size (in mm or cm)
- its shape
- its colour (there may be areas of differing pigmentation)
- its contours
- any satellite lesions within a few cm of the main melanoma
- any metastatic nodules further away from the main melanoma.

Do not forget to examine the regional lymph nodes.

You may be asked about the prognostic importance of the thickness of the melanoma, which can be measured by Clark grade I intra-epidermal) to IV (invading the subcutaneous tissues), or more usually according to the Breslow scale, which measures thickness in mm (see Table 4.2).

It is clear that the earlier a melanoma is detected and treated the better the prognosis. The golden rule is, therefore, if in doubt about a pigmented skin lesion biopsy it.

A patient with recurrent or metastatic melanoma may appear in surgical finals, since a melanoma can recur years after the original excision and metastasize widely. You should therefore ask to examine the regional lymph nodes and liver. The site of the primary lesion may be recognized by a simple scar or, commonly, a split-skin graft at the original excision site (also, look for the graft donor site, usually the thigh). Some patients may already have had regional lymph node dissection, causing a scar and also deformity of the underlying tissue. Very rarely the patient may have had an intra-ocular primary excised and hence have a glass eye.

Hence an often repeated surgical adage (with limited relevance): 'beware the patient with a large liver and a glass eye.'

Table 4.2 Breslow scale for melanoma	
Breslow thickness	5-year survival rate
< 1.5 mm	90%
1.5–3.5 mm	60%
> 3.5 mm	< 50%

Basal cell carcinoma*

Key points

- Site
- Rolled pearly edge

Basal cell carcinoma (or rodent ulcer) is usually found on the face, but occasionally on the dorsum of the hand, of elderly people with a history of exposure to sunlight. Typically, a rodent ulcer is up to 1 cm in size with a rolled, pearly edge and, usually, a central scab. You should examine for lymphadenopathy, but the rodent ulcer is, as its name suggests, locally invasive rather than metastasizing. Remember that these lesions occur in sun-damaged skin and therefore may be multiple.

Basal cell carinoma can be equally successfully treated by radiotherapy or by surgical excision.

Squamous cell carcinoma[†]

Key points

- Site
- Everted edge to ulcer
- Regional lymph nodes

Squamous cell carcinoma may be of similar appearance to basal cell carcinoma in the early stages, and it also usually occurs in sun-exposed areas of skin. However, the edge of the lesion is red, raised and everted, and the lesion may be larger than a rodent ulcer (i.e. > 1 cm). Regional lymph node metastasis may be clinically palpable. Squamous cell carcinoma may occur in the site of previous scarring ('Marjolin's ulcer').

Treatment is by radiotherapy and/or surgical excision.

Squamous cell carcinoma needs to be differentiated from kerato-acanthoma (benign, self-limiting, of infective origin) and solar (actinic) keratosis (premalignant, scaly lesion on sun-exposed skin of the elderly – treated with liquid nitrogen).

Ingrowing toenail*

Key points

- Side of the nail grows inward as a spike
- Secondary infection in overhanging skin fold

An ingrowing toenail is a classic short case for finals. Usually the great toe is affected, often in teenagers or young men. The edges of the nail bite into the adjacent pulp tissue, causing pain, erythema and often superimposed sepsis. Sometimes the result can be an impressive squidgy mess, but involvement may be limited to one border of one great toenail.

Treatment can be conservative, by trimming nails transversely rather than curving down into the corners of the nail bed, or by using cotton wool packs to lift up the nail. Surgical treatment can be by simple avulsion (but the nail often ingrows again); excision of the wedge of nail and nail bed at each affected border; or removal of the nail then excision of the nail bed deep to the cuticle (Zadek's procedure). Some surgeons use phenol to cauterize the offending nail bed.

Onychogryphosis[†]

In contrast to ingrowing toenails, this condition is usually found in the elderly and is an 'outgrowing' toenail, that may come to resemble a small horn. The lesion is said to be exacerbated by trauma or fungal infection.

It is usually treated by trimming or avulsion.

Subungual Melanoma[†]

This is an unusual form of an acral lentiginous melanoma occurring under a nail (usually the great toenail). It should form part of the differential diagnosis of any nail bed pigmentation or chronic infective process.

Dermatofibroma[†]

This is usually a single, pearly nodule within the skin. Dermato-fibromata are about 5mm in size, and typically occur on the lower limb, at the site of some previous, minor trauma.

Warts[†]

Usually occurring on the dorsum of the hand or fingers, warts (papillomata) may be an incidental finding when you examine a patient's hands. Those on the sole of the foot are known as verrucae.

Treatment involving liquid nitrogen, chemicals or surgical excision can be successful.

Fistula[†]

The opening of a fistula (a communication between one epi-thelium-lined surface and another) may be seen as a small hole, which may weep fluid or bowel content. Fistulae may occur in the neck (branchial fistula, at the lower anterior border of the ster-nomastoid muscle); on the abdominal wall (from the gastro-intestinal tract); or in the perianal area/perineum (particularly in Crohn's disease).

It may be difficult to distinguish a fistula from a blind-ended sinus, which usually results from inadequate drainage of an abscess or indicates foreign material, such as a suture, deep inside.

Pilonidal sinus[†]

A pilonidal sinus is a blind-ended pit with associated hair within. The usual location is in the natal cleft in hairy young men (and occa-sionally in young women). It can be recognized as one or several pits, usually in the midline. There may be communications or associated scarring passing superiorly and/or laterally, adjacent to a pilonidal sinus. Rarely, a pilonidal sinus may occur in the abdominal wall or, in hairdressers, in the interdigital clefts of the hands.

Definitive treatment is by excision.

Radiotherapy changes[†]

Changes in the skin due to radiotherapy can be very subtle or quite obvious. Subtle signs are the tattoo marks (each a 1–2 mm blue/

black dot) used as external markers for positioning the radiotherapy beam, which are occasionally evident on the torso or abdomen. More marked changes may be evident in the skin over the chest or head and neck, particularly if the patient was treated before the days of modern megavoltage radiotherapy. On inspection, the skin may appear pale and thickened, or quite atrophic and shiny, with telangiectasia. On palpation, the coarse or fixed skin may feel abnormal. The change from normal to treated skin may be quite abrupt at the edges of the radiation treatment fields.

Neurofibroma[§]

Rarely, a patient with neurofibromatosis may appear in surgical finals. The classical features are multiple neurofibromata (which may be of variable size) and café-au-lait skin lesions (milky-coffee-coloured areas on the skin).

Hidradenitis suppurativa[§]

In this condition, the skin in the axilla, groin or perianal area appears scarred, pitted, and frequently inflamed and abscess-bearing due to recurrent episodes of sepsis and scarring over months or years.

Treatment, if required after failed trials of antibiotics, is by excision.

Abscess/cellulitis[§]

You are unlikely to see an abscess in your exam, because abscesses are painful and therefore unlikely to be suitable for repeated examinations. However, the signs of inflammation (hot, tender, swollen, painful, with loss of function) would be present except in the case of a cold abscess (e.g. featuring in tuberculosis or actinomycosis). Examiners often ask you to speculate on the likely infecting organisms. The answer they expect is *Staphylococcus aureus* (in the case of a skin abscess), *Streptococcus* (in the case of cellulitis) or gut-derived organisms (in the case of abscesses in the perineal area).

Skin grafts[§]

Areas of skin loss which cannot be directly sutured may be closed by: a split-skin graft; a full thickness skin graft; a compound graft (such as a myocutaneous graft); or a flap. In the case of a mature split-skin graft, the underlying tissue (often muscle) is often almost visible through the graft, because of reduced skin thickness due to a lack of subcutaneous tissue. Split-skin grafts can be small postage stamp-sized pieces or extensive areas (the graft may be 'meshed' like a net to cover a large area). There should be a detectable donor site, where the donor skin has re-epithelialized, but never quite returns to a normal appearance. The donor site of a full-thickness graft may be represented simply by a linear scar or may, in turn, have been grafted with a split-skin graft. Myocutaneous flaps (latissimus dorsi, rectus abdominis, gluteal, pectoral) are unlikely to appear in finals, although they may be more likely if there is an Orthopaedic Trauma Unit, Plastic Surgery Unit or specialist Breast Unit contributing patients to finals.

Burns[§]

The severity of a burn depends on the injurious agent (usually heat), the duration of the injury, and, for thermal burns, the temperature and the speed of heat transfer (high from metal or water, lower from wood). The extent of the burns can be estimated from the size of the patient's hand (= 1% of body surface area), although this can become cumbersome – hence the 'rule of nines':

Head and neck	9%
Each upper limb	9% (× 2)
Each lower limb	9% × 2 (× 2)
Front of trunk	9% × 2
Back of trunk	9% × 2
Perineum	1%.

It is unlikely that you will be asked to examine a patient with an unhealed burn, although you may be asked about the scarring which has resulted from a full-thickness burn (with subsequent skin graft or simply healing with distorted scarring). A partial-thickness burn should heal with little residual scarring.

Others[§]

Spider naevae, port-wine stain, pyogenic granuloma, keloid scar, hypertrophic scar, keratosis or Kaposi's sarcoma may make an appearance in surgical finals. They are generally less common as short cases than the lesions mentioned above, but merit identification in an atlas of surgical signs before you go to finals, just in case. Remember though that the important point is how you examine and inspect the lesion, i.e.

- Size
- Shape
- Colour
- Position
- Consistency
- Fixation
- Associated features.

Key questions

1. What is the difference between a sebaceous cyst and a lipoma?
2. What conditions may present with lymphadenopathy?
3. Define a fistula.
4. What are the key symptoms of a melanoma?
5. What are the differences between a rodent ulcer and a squamous cell carcinoma?
6. What are the different types of skin graft?
7. How would you classify and treat burns?
8. What is a ganglion?

5

Head and neck

It is amazing how quickly you forget the anatomy that you knew so well just a few years ago! It is worth brushing up on the basic landmarks of the head and neck, and on where swellings commonly occur (Figs 5.1 and 5.2), as most head and neck cases in the exam will be swellings of some description. Stating that 'a swelling is in the submandibular triangle of the neck' will impress an examiner much more than saying 'the lump is under the chin'.

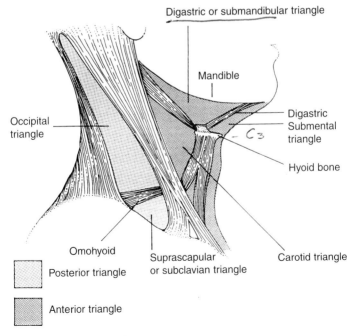

Fig. 5.1 Anatomy of the neck

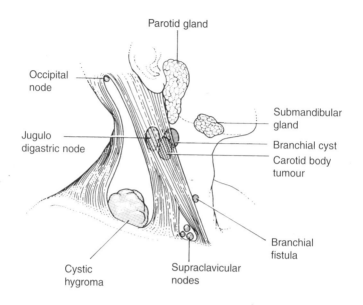

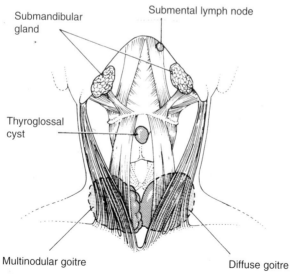

Fig. 5.2 Lesions of the neck

HISTORY

A general history of a patient with an abnormality of the head or neck should include the gender and age of the patient (some conditions are much more common in certain age groups), local symptoms and systemic symptoms. Most head and neck cancers are more common in smokers, so ask about smoking habits.

For a swelling or skin lesion, ask when it appeared; whether there has been any change in size, shape or colour; and about tenderness, redness or discharge. Has the lesion been present for a long time but changed recently? A number of developmental abnormalities may present as cystic swellings in the head and neck, usually in the second or third decades of life. For example, a branchial cyst only presents after it has become infected, or accumulated sufficient fluid to be obvious to the patient.

Systemic symptoms include sweating/fevers (e.g. in thyroid disease, tuberculosis, lymphoma, viraemia or bacteraemia); other symptoms of thyrotoxicosis (including tremor, tachycardia, agitation, weight loss); and pain in lymphomatous nodes on alcohol ingestion. These and many other features are outlined in greater detail in the appropriate sections below.

EXAMINATION

Exposure/position

Make sure you have complete exposure of the head and neck down to the clavicles, and that hair does not obscure any part of the head and neck you wish to examine. The patient will usually be sitting in a chair. A glass of water may be strategically positioned, to remind you that observing the patient swallowing can be a useful adjunct to inspection and palpation.

Inspection

Inspection is the key to identifying abnormalities in the head and neck. From a general look at the patient, gauge whether he or she shows signs of hyperthyroidism (sweating, agitation, tremor, exophthalmos) or hypothyroidism (sluggish, coarse skin, thinned hair). Are the accessory muscles of respiration being used? Looking front on to the patient, inspect from the top of the head, down the face and on to the neck and sternum: are there any visible abnormalities or scars? Then inspect each side of the head and neck in turn. Don't forget to look at the back of the neck, asking the patient to lift up their hair if necessary. Remember that lesions may lie behind the ears, or be hidden in the buccal cavity or by the tongue, so if you do not look specifically you may miss something important.

After your initial inspection, you may want to watch what happens in certain circumstances. If you suspect a midline neck swelling or thyroid swelling, ask the patient to swallow (using the glass of water if supplied). Is there any reason to suspect facial nerve palsy (e.g. a parotid tumour, or scar over the course of the facial nerve)? If so, ask the patient to show you their teeth, try to whistle and screw up their eyes (though not all three at once!), and look for weakness of one side or facial asymmetry. You may want to inspect eye movements in a patient with facial trauma (cranial nerves III and VI and the muscles they supply are particularly vulnerable to injury), or lid retraction/lid lag in someone with thyroid disease.

Point out (diplomatically, since the patient may be listening) to the examiner any skin lesions, scars, obvious lumps or swellings. Describe their

- size
- shape
- colour
- position
- consistency (palpation necessary)
- fixation to skin and/or deeper structures (palpation necessary)
- associated features (e.g. movement with swallowing).

Palpation

Palpation should focus on the abnormalities that you have spotted by a thorough inspection; aim to define the position of a lesion and elicit features such as fluctuance, which may help you come to a diagnosis. You may detect additional abnormalities (such as lymph nodes) which were not apparent on inspection.

The trachea (to test for tracheal deviation), occipital lymph nodes and sometimes midline neck lesions may be most readily palpated when standing in front of the patient. Similarly, buccal examination (wearing gloves) should be carried out when standing in front of the patient. The thyroid, parotid, anterior triangle, posterior triangle and supraclavicular structures are best palpated when standing behind the patient, who should be seated.

Specific points to consider on palpation include:

- Is the lump in the skin, subcutaneous tissues, or muscle, or is it mobile in the neck?
- Does the lump move on swallowing?
- Is the lump pulsatile, expansile or fluctuant? (Use three fingers – two to fix the lesion in place, and the third to press gently between them to test for fluctuance.)
- Can the lump be transilluminated (with a pen-torch applied to the overlying skin)? This is easier to see in a darkened room, but as an alternative, look down a tube of paper applied at one end to the skin over the illuminated lump.

Do not palpate the carotid arteries simultaneously or press too hard, in case you elicit a vagal reflex.

Percussion

Percussion in the neck may be limited to percussion over the thyroid and manubrium sternum in patients with suspected retrosternal thyroid.

Auscultation

The important structures to auscultate in the neck are the carotid vessels and the thyroid gland. A bruit in the carotid artery may be most readily heard when the patient holds his or her breath: remember to listen to both sides. A completely occluded vessel will have no flow and hence no bruit, so beware. An aortic valve murmur may be transmitted into the neck. It is said to be possible to hear a bruit over a large, hypervascular goitre – although in the exam setting this is a rare sign, listen just in case.

TYPICAL CASES

Many of the patients you are likely to encounter in surgical finals for examination of the neck will have swellings. Remember that in the case of any lump in the neck (or elsewhere) encountered in the exam (and afterwards!) you should comment on the following:

- size
- shape
- colour
- position
- fixation
- consistency
- associated features.

After inspection and palpation you should have a good idea as to what the swelling may be (see Fig. 5.2). The types of commonly encountered swellings are summarized in Table 5.1.

Table 5.1 Head and neck swellings		
	System affected	Specific lesion

Acquired	Endocrine	Thyroid*
		  – diffuse goitre
		  – solitary nodule
		  – multinodular goitre
		Carotid body tumour[§]

	Reticuloendothelial	Lymph nodes*
		  – local
		  – generalized

	Gastrointestinal	Salivary gland enlargement[†]
	Skin/subcutaneous	Sebaceous cyst* Lipoma*
Congenital		Branchial cyst* Thyroglossal cyst[†] Dermoid cyst[§] Cervical rib[§] Cystic hygroma[§]

ACQUIRED SWELLINGS

Thyroid enlargement*

History

Thyroid swellings (see Figs 5.2 and 5.3) may be associated with hyperthyroidism (e.g. in Graves' disease, toxic multinodular

Key points

- Clinical symptoms
- Nature of thyroid swelling (Fig. 5.3)
- TSH for thyroid status
- Ultrasound + Fine needle aspiration for diagnosis of thyroid swelling.

goitre); hypothyroidism (e.g. with Hashimoto's thyroiditis, iodine deficiency, drugs including lithium) or the euthyroid state (e.g. with physiological goitre, multinodular goitre, solitary nodules). It is important to ask for clues about the state of the patient's thyroid, such as sweating, agitation, tremor, tachycardia or atrial fibrillation (which occur with hyperthyroidism) and pretibial myxoedema, increasing lethargy, cold intolerance, weight gain and voice changes (which occur with hypothyroidism).

In addition to being noted as a swelling, a large (and/or retrosternal) goitre can cause tracheal compression (with stridor), dysphonia and even dysphagia. An anaplastic carcinoma of the thyroid may cause a recurrent laryngeal nerve palsy, resulting in a hoarse voice and bovine cough. Goitres are usually painless, but pain does occur with subacute thyroiditis (de Quervain's), haemorrhage into a cyst, rapidly enlarging anaplastic carcinomas and, occasionally, Hashimoto's thyroiditis.

Examination

Examination of the thyroid follows the familiar scheme of inspection, palpation, percussion and auscultation, following which you will have some idea as to the likely diagnosis (Fig. 5.3). During the examination, bear in mind the possible diagnoses associated with each of multinodular goitre, diffuse enlargement and solitary nodules. Apparently diffuse enlargement suggests Graves' disease, anaplastic carcinoma, simple (deficiency) goitre, sarcoidosis, or (if tender) thyroiditis. A single nodule suggests a simple cyst, a benign adenoma, follicular or papillary carcinoma.

With the patient's neck and shoulders adequately exposed, inspect from the front and sides. Is there a single lump, or is there a diffuse swelling? Decide on the position of the lump, and look for

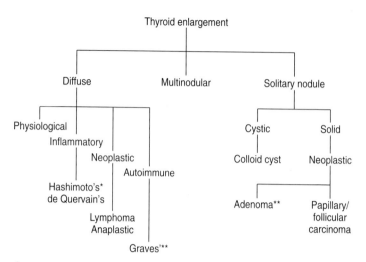

Fig. 5.3 Thyroid swellings

movement with swallowing – a thyroid lump moves up, then down, as the patient swallows, due to the envelopment of the thyroid gland in the pretracheal fascia. Consider the features applicable to any lump. The shape of a thyroid swelling will be that of a diffuse enlargement, a unilobular enlargement or a single nodule, and its size (in cm) should be measured. Remember to inspect (and palpate) for associated cervical lymph nodes, or the attachment of the goitre to local structures. If given the opportunity, look for lid lag, ophthalmoplegia, and altered reflexes. Features associated with an enlarged thyroid may include regional lymph node enlargement or a bruit.

Stand behind the patient to palpate the thyroid, and ask the patient to swallow: this is when a glass of water may be useful (try to swallow several times when *you* are dry-mouthed and nervous). The gland's consistency is important – hard, woody glands are associated with either malignancy or thyroiditis, and fixation to the trachea indicates malignancy.

Percuss (over the sternum for a retrosternal goitre).

Auscultate (with the patient holding his or her breath) for the bruit of a hyperdynamic thyroid blood flow, occasionally found in Graves' disease.

Investigation

Blood tests

- Thyroid stimulating hormone (TSH) – to distinguish between biochemically hyperthyroid patients (low TSH) and thyroid failure (high TSH);
  this can be supplemented with Triiodothyronine (T3)/thyroxine (T4)
- Circulating antibodies – for Hashimoto's or Graves' disease
- Calcitonin – for medullary thyroid cancer (also used to detect early cases of multiple endocrine neoplasia).

Radiology

- Chest radiograph – for a soft tissue mass in the upper mediastinum
- Thoracic outlet views – for a suspected retrosternal thyroid
- Ultrasound scanning – can determine whether a palpable thyroid lump is cystic or solid, and whether it is solitary or multiple
- Radionuclide scanning – can identify whether thyroid lesions are 'hot' (benign) or 'cold' (potentially malignant). Confusingly, thyroid metastases may also show up as hot nodules on scanning, because the uptake of isotope by the metastasis is greater than by the surrounding normal tissue.

Other investigations   A fine needle can be used to obtain cells from cystic or solid lesions by aspiration for cytology.

Ultrasound visualisation of a thyroid swelling combined with fine needle aspiration cytology (FNAC) have become the investigations of choice in expert centres.

Treatment

The treatment of thyroid disease may be conservative (for benign, minimally enlarged, euthyroid goitre), medical (oral thyroxine to correct hypothyroidism), radiotherapy (radioiodine for hyperthyroidism) or surgery (thyroid lobectomy, subtotal thyroidectomy, or total thyroidectomy, depending on the condition being treated).

The complications of surgery (though rare) include recurrent laryngeal nerve palsy, superior laryngeal nerve palsy, hypocalcaemia (transient, but may be severe), tracheal compression due to a haematoma, or a thyroid storm).

Cervical nodes*

Key points

- Symptoms and number and distribution of nodes suggest the most useful investigation(s) and likely diagnosis

History

Ask about the position and duration of the swelling(s), and any related pain. Enquire about systemic symptoms, e.g. sweating (sometimes at night), pain in the nodes on alcohol ingestion (in the case of lymphoma), and whether there is enlargement of other lymph node groups. Has there been any intraoral disease process such as tooth decay, or discharge from the lump(s) into the mouth or to the skin? Ask whether there have been any serious medical illnesses or surgical operations elsewhere in the past (thinking particularly of metastatic disease). Ask whether there has been any contact with animals or any foreign travel. Bear in mind the age and racial origin of the patient, which may point you towards the more likely diagnoses.

Examination

Expose the patient's head and neck, and position him or her so as to be comfortable (usually seated) and so that you can examine him or her with ease.

Note whether there are any general features of disease (such as jaundice, cachexia), or heavily nicotine-stained fingers. Remember that inspection, then palpation, should enable you to comment on the position and size of enlarged lymph nodes; their shape; whether they are single, multiple or matted to each other; any fixation of the glands to the overlying skin, adjacent structures, underlying muscle or each other; their consistency (soft/rubbery/hard); the colour of the overlying skin; and whether there are associated lesions such as generalized lymphadenopathy or intraoral lesions. Inspection of the neck should guide you to the principal node groups involved and to any skin tethering (e.g. at the site of a tuberculous node sinus). Always remember to inspect areas from which a lymph node may be draining – look in the mouth to see if the submental lymph node you have just identified is due to intraoral sepsis or to intraoral carcinoma.

Palpation should be performed systematically. Stand behind the seated patient and use the pulps of your fingers to gently palpate the left and right sides simultaneously (so that you can compare them as you go along), starting anteriorly at the chin and passing posteriorly beneath the mandible. Patients often try to help you by lifting their chin, but as this has the opposite effect, you may need to remind them to drop the chin. With gentle rotating movements of your finger pulps, you should palpate even quite small nodes. At the angle of the mandible, pass inferiorly down the anterior border of sternomastoid, palpating the anterior triangle nodes. Return to the angle of the mandible and palpate the preauricular (parotid) and retroauricular regions. Then move your hands inferiorly to examine the posterior triangle, and further inferiorly down to the supraclavicular fossa and then the infraclavicular fossa, before finally checking the occipital nodes. Much is made in exams of Troisier's sign, a palpable lymph node in the left supraclavicular fossa (Virchow's node). It is unusual to find this node in isolation.

Investigation

Blood tests   A full blood count, blood film and erythrocyte sedimentation rate (ESR) should be obtained. In certain circumstances it may be appropriate to check the serum for viral titres (e.g. Epstein – Barr antibodies, or HIV status after counselling) and other organisms.

Radiology   A chest radiograph may confirm the clinical diagnosis, for example by revealing hilar nodes, the Ghon focus of tuberculosis, bronchogenic carcinoma or secondary malignancy. Ultrasound scanning may differentiate nodes from other neck lumps.

Other investigations   A full examination of the nasopharynx, including laryngoscopy and possibly endoscopic examination of the upper gastrointestinal tract, should also be considered. Fine needle aspiration cytology and/or biopsy may provide a definitive answer as to what pathological process underlies the lymphadenopathy.

Salivary glands[†]

Key points

- The history often suggests the likely diagnosis
- Tumours usually involve the parotid gland
- Calculi usually occur in the submandibular gland
- Ultrasound (± fine needle aspiration) can secure the diagnosis

There are three major pairs of salivary glands (parotid, submandibular and sublingual), and numerous unnamed glands throughout the oral mucosa. Tumours and stones generally affect a single major gland, but viral illness and autoimmune disease may affect several or all of the glands. The features of the most commonly encountered salivary gland swellings are listed in Table 5.2.

History

The duration of the swelling, whether it is unilateral or bilateral and whether the swelling increases with salivary stimulation can all hint at the pathological process involved. The latter symptom, which suggests a stone in the duct, may be associated with a gush of metallic-tasting salivary fluid as the stone falls back. Pain usually suggests an inflammatory process – the parotid in particular is invested in a dense cervical fascia, and acute enlargement can be extremely painful.

Examination

With the patient suitably positioned and adequately exposed, visual inspection may well hint at the diagnosis, or at least suggest which gland is involved. The parotid gland is bilateral (so remember to compare the two sides), and comprises two parts: the preauricular and the retromandibular (deep to the angle of the jaw). The former is readily palpable, particularly when enlarged by tumour, by an obstructing stone or by an inflammatory process (e.g. infection by mumps virus, which may cause unilateral or bilateral swelling). Of tumours, 80% occur in the parotid, and 15% in the submandibular gland; while 80% of obstructing stones occur in the submandibular gland, and 20% in the parotid. The deep part of the parotid gland may be difficult to distinguish from the submandibular gland or from cervical lymph nodes on clinical

Table 5.2   Salivary gland swellings

Type of lesion	Features
Neoplastic	
Pleomorphic adenomas	Most commonly in parotid Benign/slow growth, but local recurrence if enucleated Patients usually < 50 years of age
Adenolymphoma	Often soft/partially cystic Benign/slow growing Patients usually > 50 years of age
Anaplastic carcinoma	Fast growing Hard and woody Invades locally VIIth cranial nerve palsy Regional lymphadenopathy Retrotonsillar enlargement
Salivary calculi	Submandibular gland most commonly involved Intermittent swelling Pain
Inflammatory	
Viral	
– Mumps	Usually bilateral, but occasionally unilateral Painful Prodromal illness
Autoimmune	Associated with dry mouth/eyes Frequently bilateral Associated with connective tissue disease, e.g. Siögren's syndrome, Mikulicz's syndrome
Acute parotitis	Associated with poor oral hygiene
Sialectasis	
Sarcoidosis	

examination, but can be affected by the same disease processes as can affect the superficial parotid. Occasionally a parotid tumour will enlarge into the retrotonsillar space, so remember to examine inside the mouth. While looking in the mouth, visualize the parotid duct orifice (in the cheek opposite the upper second molar) and the submandibular duct opening (on the floor of the mouth adjacent to the frenulum of the tongue) – you may see a stone. Test the VIIth cranial nerve for facial nerve palsy. The facial nerve runs through the parotid gland and is in danger of transection during surgical exploration. Parotid tumours may also cause a VIIth nerve paralysis. The cervical branch of the facial nerve is closely applied to the submandibular gland, and may be damaged in surgical excision of this gland.

Palpate the parotid and submandibular glands. An abnormal submandibular gland should be readily palpable if the patient relaxes the chin inferiorly. Don't forget that intraoral examination (wearing gloves), to palpate the submandibular ducts and glands and the parotid duct, is an important part of the examination of the salivary glands: say so to your examiner. After palpation of the glands, feel for regional nodal enlargement.

Investigation

Blood tests In addition to basic haematology, biochemical and immunological studies (for viral infection or manifestations of immunological systemic disease such as rheumatoid arthritis).

Radiology Ultrasound scanning may be helpful to differentiate between salivary glands and other structures in the neck. If stones in the submandibular glands are suspected, plain radiology of the floor of the mouth may be supplemented by sialograms (for which radioopaque dye is injected via a cannula into the salivary duct to demonstrate ectatic ducts and/or obstruction).

Other investigations Fine needle aspiration cytology (FNAC) or core biopsy (under local anaesthetic) have their advocates, and may confirm the diagnosis.

Carotid body tumour[§]

This is a firm lump (which, together with the macroscopic appearance on sectioning, gives the alternative name, 'potato tumour') in the course of the carotid artery. Such tumours may be bilateral and can be associated with blackouts or transient ischaemic episodes.

CONGENITAL SWELLINGS

Branchial cyst[†]

A branchial cyst develops because of a failure of fusion of the embryonic second and third branchial arches. It is unusual for a cyst to present before adolescence, when it is seen as a smooth rubbery swelling, bulging forwards from deep to the anterior border of the middle third of sternomastoid. Occasionally there is a branchial fistula (a communication between two epithelium-lined surfaces) running between the tonsillar fossa and the skin at the anterior border of sternomastoid, at the junction of its middle and lower third (where it can be hidden behind clothing if the neck is not adequately exposed).

Thyroglossal cyst[†]

This is a remnant of the thyroglossal duct, from which the thyroid gland develops. A thyroglossal cyst is usually a smooth, rounded swelling located in the midline between the thyroid isthmus and the hyoid bone. It is non-tender (unless infected) and is rubbery in consistency. It moves upwards then downwards when the patient swallows, because of the attachment of the pretracheal fascia.

Excision may necessitate removal of the whole thyroglossal duct, which originates at the foramen caecum (at the junction of the anterior two-thirds and posterior third of the tongue) and takes a convoluted course around the hyoid bone down to the isthmus of the thyroid.

Dermoid cyst[§]

Dermoid cysts on the head or neck are usually inclusion cysts, resulting from the sequestration of dermal cells at the site of fusion of embryonic clefts and sinuses. They present as smooth, mobile cutaneous swellings, in the region of the supraorbital ridge (external angular dermoid cyst) or in the midline at the base of the nose or inferior to the chin (submental dermoid cyst). An implantation dermoid cyst is caused by the traumatic implantation of skin, and usually occurs elsewhere, such as on the hands or feet.

Cervical rib[§]

A cervical rib may be visible as a lump superior to the clavicle, with a palpable subclavian artery. The symptoms are neurological (T1 and C8 pain and weakness) or, rarely, vascular (e.g. rest pain or Raynaud's phenomenon – pallor and pain in the digits followed by cyanosis, then rubor as the phenomenon relents), due to pressure by the cervical rib on the subclavian artery.

Cystic hygroma[§]

A cystic hygroma is a collection of dilated lymphatic channels, found at the base of the posterior triangle (related to the thoracic duct, if on the left side of the neck). A cystic hygroma usually presents in children as a soft, fluctuant, compressible lump, which may be large enough to occupy the base of the posterior triangle. This position is characteristic, and the diagnosis is usually clinched by transillumination. A cystic hygroma is said to be 'brilliantly transilluminable'.

Skin lesions on the head and neck

History

It is important to ask about both the patient's age and the history of a lump. Patients with sebaceous cysts or Peutz–Jeghers syndrome may be young; patients with skin malignancy are often, but not exclusively, elderly. Changes in the size, shape and colour of a lesion (particularly if a melanoma is suspected), and episodes of swelling, pain and discharge should all be explored with the patient. Prolonged exposure to sunlight (what is/was the patient's occupation?) may be aetiological in skin malignancy of the head or neck.

Examination

Once again, follow the exposure, inspection, palpation (. . . percussion, auscultation) scheme.

Skin lesions occur on the head and neck, just as elsewhere on the body, and can be within the skin (e.g. sebaceous cyst, basal cell carcinoma, squamous cell carcinoma, melanoma) or in the subcutaneous tissues (e.g. lipoma, neuroma, fibroma). Typical skin lesions of the head and neck (covered in more detail in Ch. 4) include:

- sebaceous cyst[*] (in the skin, has a punctum)
- lipoma[*] (subcutaneous, appears fluctuant)
- melanoma[*] (change in size, shape, or colour)
- basal cell carcinoma[*] (a rolled pearly edge, typically develops over the midface)
- squamous cell carcinoma[†] (remember neck nodes).

Also, beware of scarring from burns, surgery or radiotherapy (often with telangiectasis in skin which is thin and shiny or coarse and thickened). Remember that squamous carcinoma can arise in scar tissue (when it is called a Marjolin's ulcer).

Despite their rarity in the real world, the perioral freckles of Peutz–Jeghers syndrome (which also comprises multiple benign polyps in the small bowel) and the telangiectasia around the mouth, lips and gums in hereditary haemorrhagic telangiectasia (associated also with gastrointestinal bleeding) are such classical symptoms that they can be used for spot diagnoses.

A range of 'medical' conditions may also manifest themselves on the skin of the head and neck, including jaundice, anaemia, psoriasis, the malar flush of mitral valve disease, herpes zoster, and xanthelasma.

Eye signs

In surgical finals, eye signs of disease elsewhere are usually due to a nerve palsy (usually IIIrd nerve, rarely VIth nerve, and occasionally Horner's syndrome) or are related to thyroid disease (e.g. lid lag, exophthalmos, ophthalmoplegia).

History

Symptoms of hyperthyroidism, head or facial trauma, or smoking (e.g. Pancoast's syndrome) may give a hint as to the condition responsible for the eye signs. Pancoast's syndrome is the spectrum of symptoms and signs caused by a bronchogenic carcinoma at the apex of the lung (sometimes called a Pancoast's (bronchogenic) carcinoma) including severe pain (which may radiate down the arm), Horner's syndrome and rib erosion.

Examination

Initial inspection may enable you to spot the diagnosis in some cases, e.g. the exophthalmos of thyrotoxicosis; ipsilateral miosis and ptosis in Horner's syndrome (enophthalmos and the ipsilateral loss of sweating of the face may be less obvious); IIIrd nerve palsy (ipsilateral large pupil, ptosis, downward and outward gaze); subconjunctival haemorrhage. Less immediately apparent features (but common and still worthy of mention to your examiner) include arcus senilis and xanthelasmata.

Beware of the glass eye: you would not be the first exam candidate to be caught out. A glass eye may be a very good colour match compared with the normal eye, but does not have the full range of movement. Also, there will be no pupillary reflex to light, or accommodation!

Visual field assessment, fundoscopy and detailed examination of the cranial nerves are usually reserved for the medical part of final exams, or postgraduate exams.

Investigation

It may be appropriate to mention laboratory tests for thyroid disease, lipid/cholesterol levels, diabetes or other metabolic disorders, depending on your clinical findings.

A chest radiograph may detect a lesion causing Horner's syndrome (e.g. ipsilateral Horner's syndrome caused by invasion of the cervical sympathetic plexus due to carcinoma of the bronchus).

Facial nerve palsy[§]

Facial (VIIth) nerve palsy can be due to either a lower motor neurone lesion (typically secondary to trauma, surgery to the parotid, tumour of the parotid or Bell's palsy) or an upper motor neurone lesion (in which case the frontalis muscle is spared due to bilateral cortical representation). A lower motor neurone lesion may only affect the branches transected (test the orbicularis oris, orbicularis oculi and frontalis muscles).

Cushingoid facies*

A Cushingoid facies in surgical finals is usually iatrogenic. Patients receiving steroids for chronic inflammatory disease (e.g. arthritis, inflammatory bowel disease), immunosuppression or auto-immune disease may develop Cushingoid features – they are rarely due to endogenous excess steroid production.

Signs of this condition include a moon face with red rounded cheeks, facial hirsutism, easily bruised, fragile skin, striae (e.g. on the abdominal wall and thighs), proximal myopathy, and buffalo hump (which may be accentuated by osteoporotic collapse of the spine).

Miscellaneous

Occasionally in exams you may be asked to comment on a central line or a tracheostomy.

Central venous lines*

A central venous line is inserted either to allow monitoring of central venous pressure or to allow venous access – most commonly for parenteral nutrition or chemotherapy. The tip of the line itself should lie in the superior vena cava at the junction with the right atrium, where it should be visible on a chest radiograph. A venous line is a potential portal for infection (infection may be reduced by inserting the line through a skin tunnel), so the line should always be handled with an aseptic technique.

The complications associated with a central line relate firstly to its insertion and secondly to its management. During insertion it is possible to damage anatomically related structures in the neck, i.e. the apex of the lung/pleura, the subclavian artery, branches of the brachial plexus or even the thoracic duct (on the left side): pneumothorax and haemothorax are worth remembering. It is also possible to cause an air embolism, or embolism of the tip of the line if it is sheared off during insertion. If the line is in so far that it lies within the atrium, it may precipitate dysrhythmias. Longer term complications are usually related to infection of the line, but it is possible for the tip of the line to erode the vascular structures or to precipitate a subclavian thrombosis. The complications of TPN (total parenteral nutrition) therapy (electrolyte imbalance, hyperosmolarity, hyperammonaemia, metal ion deficiency) or chemotherapy may occur.

Tracheostomy§

A tracheostomy tube is inserted through the upper two tracheal cartilages, inferior to the cricoid cartilage, to allow access to the airway for ventilation, reduce respiratory dead space and allow bronchial suction. It is most often performed electively in patients who require prolonged ventilation, as it is easier to manage and less traumatic than an orotracheal tube, which would pass through the vocal cords. Patients who have undergone a laryngectomy will have a permanent tracheostomy. The principal complications of a tracheostomy are bleeding or airway obstruction, particularly at the time of insertion; drying of bronchial secretions (if the inspired air is not humidified), which may lead to pulmonary collapse or blockage of the tracheostomy; damage to the tracheal wall (from the cuff on the tracheostomy tube), with late stenosis; displacement of the tube into the neck (with resultant surgical emphysema); or the tube may fall out completely.

Key questions

1. What are the causes of the following types of thyroid enlargement:
   - single nodule? *STA*
   - multinodular? *MNL*
   - diffuse? *Graves*
2. What are the causes of enlargement of the parotid gland and of the submandibular gland? *⇒ Stone*
3. What are the causes of cervical lymphadenopathy:
   - limited to the neck? *lympma*
   - as part of a systemic lymphadenopathy? *Lympm, mets*
4. What congenital swellings can occur and where are they sited in the head and neck? *Thyroglossal cyst, Cystic hygroma.*
5. What are the features of the following:
   - a sebaceous cyst? *punctum*
   - a lipoma? *Subcutaneous, sr*
   - a basal cell carcinoma?
   - a squamous cell carcinoma? *Metastasis*
   - a malignant melanoma?
6. What are the causes of a VIIth nerve lesion:
   - upper motor neurone? *Stroke, MS,*
   - lower motor neurone?
7. What are the indications for and complications of the following:
   - a tracheostomy?
   - a central venous line?

6

Chest

In surgical exams you are less likely to be asked to examine the cardiac or respiratory systems in detail than in medical finals. However, surgically relevant features such as signs of cardiac, pulmonary or gastro-oesophageal surgery and signs of surgically important pulmonary or pleural disease do form part of surgical finals. You should remember that significant cardiopulmonary disease may well limit the treatment options in certain patients: this may be a central point in the discussion following your long case. For example, you may be faced with a patient who gives a typical history of biliary colic but who also has severe chronic obstructive pulmonary disease: the examiner may well quiz you on the risks of surgery and on how potential problems in this patient could be averted.

The American Society of Anesthesiologists (ASA) has developed a grading system which indicates, on the basis of the severity of pre-existing disease (often cardiorespiratory), a patient's risk of death as a result of surgery. In simplified form:

- ASA1 – normal
- ASA2 – mild-moderate systemic disturbance
- ASA3 – severe systemic disturbance
- ASA4 – life-threatening systemic disorder
- ASA5 – moribund patient with little chance of survival.

You may be asked to examine the chest of a patient in surgical finals: this usually means just that. There is a subtle distinction between being asked to examine the chest and being asked to examine the respiratory system or cardiovascular system (in which case you should start with the hands!), so make sure you listen to what your examiner asks.

HISTORY

The principal respiratory symptoms are cough, sputum, haemoptysis, breathlessness, chest pain and wheeze. The main cardiac symptoms are chest pain, breathlessness, ankle swelling and palpitations. These symptoms may all be significant in assessing a patient's suitability for surgery and if any are present, determine their severity. Does the patient get breathless when running for a bus, walking briskly or walking short distances, or on minimal exertion such as dressing?

Symptoms of diseases of the respiratory system relevant to surgical practice include sharp (pleuritic) chest pain, shortness of breath and haemoptysis. These can be caused by infections (e.g. pneumonia, empyema, bronchiectasis, tuberculosis); tumours (e.g. primary lung carcinoma, secondaries); vascular problems (e.g. pulmonary infarction/embolism, heart failure) or trauma (e.g. fractured ribs). Ask about any history of thoracic surgery (e.g. lung or pleural resection, surgical pneumothorax for anti-tubercle surgery), midline sternotomy (for a coronary artery bypass graft (CABG) or other cardiac procedures) or left thoracotomy (for mitral valve replacement).

EXAMINATION

Think, as you examine the chest, what might be the underlying problem. Is there a unilateral condition (e.g. pleural effusion, lobar pneumonia)? Is there a bilateral condition (e.g. bilateral crepitations of heart failure)? Are there any clues? There may be signs of intrathoracic disease elsewhere, particularly in the hands (e.g. finger clubbing, palmar erythema, radial pulse); head and neck (e.g. lymph nodes, jugular venous pressure); abdomen (e.g. liver) and lower limbs (e.g. peripheral oedema).

Exposure/position

Expose the torso so that it can be fully examined. For a chest examination, the traditional position for the patient is sitting propped up on pillows at a 45-degree angle. Alternatively, you may be presented with a patient sitting in a chair. When examining the chest, compare right with left and front with back.

Inspection

Inspection of the chest should include the use of your ears for the tell-tale clicking of a prosthetic heart valve (usually mitral or aortic). Look for and comment on the presence of any deformities (e.g. kyphoscoliosis) or surgical scars. There may also be evidence of other surgical procedures, for example central, feeding or chemotherapy lines, chest drains or cardiac pacemaker (though all of these are sometimes inserted by physicians).

Assess the patient's respiratory rate and look for signs of laboured breathing, including the use of the accessory respiratory muscles, the intercostal muscles being drawn in and chest expansion. With the patient propped up at 45°, look for the jugular venous pulse wave and the height (pressure) of the filled vein. Look for signs of superior vena cava obstruction – swelling of the conjunctivae, face, neck and upper limbs; visible collateral veins and prominent jugular veins. Check the sputum pot for coloured sputum and the presence of blood.

Palpation

Palpation should begin by examining the trachea for deviation to one side (pushed by a growth or intrapleural expansion, or pulled as a result of collapse or contraction to the side of the disease process). Test for chest expansion, both anteriorly and posteriorly – poor expansion is a sign of a disease process on that side of the chest (bilateral in chronic obstructive airways disease). Feel for vocal fremitus.

Percussion

Percuss down each rib space (don't forget the apices or the midaxillary line, and remember that the liver lies on the right-hand side, up to the fourth intercostal space). Where does the percussion note change from resonant to dull?

Auscultation

After checking the tracheal position, testing for expansion and percussing the chest, you should have some idea of whether you are going to find a unilateral or bilateral abnormality when you listen to the lung fields. Feel for the apex beat, which may be displaced due to intrathoracic disease from its position of the fifth intercostal space in the midclavicular line.

Auscultate for breath sounds using the bell of the stethoscope, listening for crackles (fine/coarse/clear with coughing?), bronchial breathing and, where indicated, whispering pectoriloquy (ask the patient to say 1–1–1). You may hear bowel sounds when you examine the chest of a surgical patient, due to a hiatus hernia or following gastro-oesophageal resection and reconstruction.

INVESTIGATION

In addition to the basic biochemical and haematological investigations, chest radiology (posterior/anterior film and lateral view) plays a particularly important role in confirming the clinical diagnosis (See Radiology chapter 13).

Spirometry, to measure forced expiratory volume in one second (FEV_1), forced vital capacity (FVC) and the FEV_1/FVC ratio, can be useful for comparing a patient's pulmonary function with that expected for their height and gender. Arterial blood gas measurement will indicate the arterial Po_2 and Pco_2 and any acid/base imbalances.

Do not forget that sputum cytology, needle aspiration of an effusion and bronchoscopy may contribute useful information about pulmonary or pleural diseases. An ECG, echocardiography and radiological imaging (e.g. after cardiac catheterization) may be useful in the diagnosis of cardiac disease.

TYPICAL CASES

Pleural effusion*

Key points

- Stony dull percussion note and absent breath sounds over effusion
- Chest radiographs for diagnosis
- Aspiration for diagnosis

History

The history should include details of cardiac and respiratory symptoms and treatment, and enquiries about previous medical conditions (such as rheumatic fever) and surgical operations, particularly for cancer. The lungs and pleurae are favoured sites for metastatic disease from epithelial cancers.

Examination

On inspection, the patient may look unwell (e.g. cachectic due to cancer). There may be signs of a previous aspiration or chest drainage procedure (e.g. bruising, a needle puncture or an Elastoplast), and chest expansion may be diminished on the affected side. Palpation may reveal reduced expansion, and on percussion there may be a stony, dull percussion note over the effusion (large unilateral effusions are easier to detect than small bilateral effusions). On auscultation, breath sounds should be absent over the effusion, although there may be bronchial breathing at the top of the effusion.

Investigation

A standard PA (posteroanterior) chest radiograph, supplemented by a lateral view, should confirm the presence of a pleural effusion by demonstrating loss of the costophrenic angle on the affected side and a homogeneous shadowing with a border which is concave upwards. Aspiration of the pleural cavity (under ultrasound guidance if it is a small effusion) enables cytological, biochemical and bacteriological analysis of the fluid, which may be straw-coloured or blood-stained. The protein content of the aspirate will indicate whether this is an exudate or a transudate.

Diagnosis

If you are asked 'What are likely causes of a pleural effusion?', start with the commonest and therefore the most likely diagnosis (Fig.6.1). In surgical finals, exudates (protein > 30 g/l) are more common than transudates. Exudates may be due to primary tumours (e.g. bronchogenic carcinoma, mesothelioma); secondary tumours (e.g. a malignant pleural effusion due to breast, lung, ovarian or gastrointestinal cancer); infection within the chest (e.g. pneumonia, tuberculosis) or, rarely, to vascular lesions such as

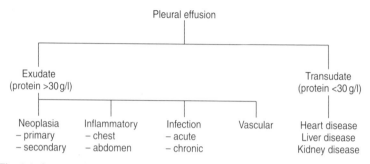

Fig. 6.1 Causes of pleural effusion

pulmonary emboli. Exudates may also be secondary to intra-abdominal inflammation or sepsis (e.g. pancreatitis, subphrenic abscess). A transudate (protein < 30 g/l) suggests a medical cause, particularly heart failure, cirrhosis or nephrotic syndrome.

Bronchogenic carcinoma[†]

Although lung cancers are depressingly common in clinical practice, you are far more likely to encounter one in your medical than in your surgical exams. This diagnosis should be considered for patients who are middle-aged or older and have haemoptysis or a persistent cough – particularly if they are smokers. Other clinical presentations may indicate more advanced disease, for example involving malignant pleural effusions or lymph node metastases. A bovine cough may be due to compression of the left recurrent laryngeal nerve by a hilar tumour. An unusual presentation occurs when an apical tumour (which may be visible on the chest radiograph) erodes into the first rib, causing pain and weakness in the arm in association with unilateral ptosis, miosis, enophthalmos and hypohydrosis (Horner's syndrome); this combination of tumour and Horner's syndrome is known as Pancoast's syndrome.

History

If you suspect a lung tumour, ask the patient about occupation, previous lung disease and smoking.

Examination

On inspection, look for signs which may support your diagnosis: nicotine-stained fingers, finger clubbing, signs of cachexia and, more rarely, superior vena cava obstruction due to mediastinal disease. Listen for evidence of recurrent laryngeal nerve paralysis. On palpation, percussion and auscultation, look for tracheal deviation and chest signs indicating a pleural effusion or pulmonary collapse. Palpate for cervical lymph nodes, rib metastases and hepatomegaly due to metastatic disease.

Investigation

As in the case of most chest problems, along with basic haematology, PA and lateral chest radiographs, sputum cytology and bronchoscopy (with brushings, lavage and/or biopsy) should aim to establish the diagnosis.

Heart valves[†]

Most open cardiac surgery involves coronary artery bypass grafting (CABG) or valve replacement, although less invasive methods, particularly those practised by radiologists and cardiologists, have become increasingly common. Patients who have or are due to undergo heart surgery generally fall into one of two groups: young patients who have congenital cardiac problems or have suffered infective endocarditis with valve destruction, and older patients in whom the predominant underlying pathology is degenerative vascular disease and/or a past history of rheumatic fever.

History

Ask direct questions about the patient's current and past cardiac symptoms, including breathlessness, angina, symptoms of peripheral vascular disease, and strokes(s). Ask about current and previous medications. Also ask specific questions about rheumatic fever, hypertension, myocardial infarction and investigative procedures. Most patients have had echocardiography (ultrasound scanning of the heart, including the valves, for structure and function) or coronary and/or cardiac angiography (performed through percutaneous puncture of the femoral artery prior to surgery), and may be quite knowledgeable about their investigations and the results. Patients usually also know the type of valve (mechanical or porcine graft) which has been used, and may be able to state the make.

Examination

Estimate the patient's age and assess his or her general health: a fat, elderly patient is unlikely to have significant congenital heart disease, but is likely to have ischaemic heart disease or perhaps rheumatic heart disease.

The upper half of the patient's body should be exposed, and traditionally the patient is examined sitting propped up at 45°. Inspection of the torso from the front and sides will reveal surgical scars such as a midline sternotomy scar (usually indicating CABG), often accompanied by scars in the epigastrium, from drainage tubes. The left thoracic approach for valve surgery and associated drain sites are usually clearly visible – if you take the trouble to inspect the left chest wall! While inspecting, listen for the rhythmic clicking of a prosthetic valve and if you hear it, comment on it to the examiner. During inspection you may see the jugular venous pressure (with the patient sitting propped up at 45°), and the apex beat may be visible.

Prior to auscultation, take the patient's hand and feel the pulse for rate, rhythm, and character. Then examine for the JVP (if not already visible), systolic and diastolic blood pressures, apex beat (the fifth intercostal space in the midclavicular line) and valvular thrills.

Auscultation begins before you use the stethoscope: that irritating click (which may be regular or irregular) may turn out to be the patient's heart valve, not someone's watch! Any mechanical prosthetic valve will probably have a deafening click when you listen with a stethoscope. Use the diaphragm of the stethoscope to auscultate the heart except when seeking a mitral stenotic murmur. Cardiac murmurs are traditionally medical territory, but for a surgeon's guide to the common ones see Table 6.1.

Investigation

In addition to urine testing (for glucose) and basic haematology and biochemistry, the mainstays of cardiology are the ECG and, primarily, echocardiography (which can detect many abnormalities in the structure and function of the heart, including the valves).

Chest radiographs (PA and lateral) can be valuable for revealing cardiac size, shape and outline as well as lung field and pleural abnormalities. More advanced imaging (e.g. involving cardiac

Table 6.1 Cardiac murmurs	
Condition	Type of murmur
Aortic stenosis	Ejection systolic murmur Radiates to carotids
Aortic regurgitation	Early diastolic murmur Left sternal edge Best heard with the patient leaning forward, on expiration
Mitral stenosis	Mid-diastolic murmur At apex
Mitral regurgitation	Pansystolic murmur At apex Radiates to axilla Best heard with the patient in the left lateral position, using the bell of the stethoscope

catheterization, coronary angiography, radioisotope scanning for function) may be considered if available.

Chest drains[†]

A patient with a chest drain may show up in finals. The first thing you have to do is to recognize that it is a chest drain. You may think that this sounds simple, but it is surprising what people have thought chest drains are in the heat of an exam. A chest drain comes from an intercostal space and goes to a collecting bottle, with the end of the tube beneath the surface of the fluid (Fig. 6.2). When the patient coughs or breathes, the fluid within the drainage tube should move with the changing intrapleural pressure. If there is bubbling when the patient exhales, there is a persisting pneumothorax.

If you are confronted with a chest drain, you will almost certainly be asked 'How should this be connected up?' The answer is that the end of the drainage tube must be under the surface of the fluid in the collecting bottle, and the bottle must be kept below the drainage site. However, one-way valve systems exist, which have the same effect. If the patient has to be moved, the tube should be double-clamped close to the patient in case it becomes detached or fluid syphons into the patient (if the bottle is placed higher than the patient).

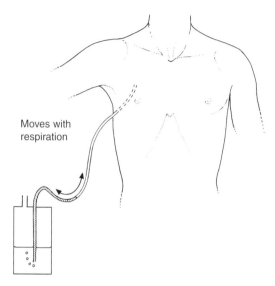

Moves with
respiration

Fig. 6.2 Chest drain

Chest drains may be inserted to drain air (e.g. in pneumothorax), fluid (e.g. in pleural effusion), pus (e.g. in empyema) or
blood (e.g. in haemothorax) (see Table 6.2).

Table 6.2 Positioning and use of chest drains	
Condition	Position/purpose of chest drain
Pleural effusion	Usually inserted in the most gravity-dependent part of the pleural space, usually in the midaxillary line
Pneumothorax	Usually in the midclavicular line, in the second intercostal space. If there is bubbling, low pressure suction may be needed
Postoperative	Post-thoracotomy, one or two chest drains are usually inserted to prevent air or fluid collections
Empyema	Site of drain will depend on that of the collection. If pus is not draining, a rib resection may be needed
Trauma	Blood and/or air in the pleural cavity should be drained via the fifth intercostal space in the midaxillary line

Pneumonectomy[§]

Pneumonectomy or pulmonary lobectomy is usually performed either for benign, inflammatory pulmonary conditions (e.g. bronchiectasis, tuberculosis) or for malignancy (usually primary carcinoma of the lung, but sometimes isolated lung metastases).

History

Given the opportunity, the patient will often help considerably by telling you what operation has been done. The history should include particular attention to the drugs or chemotherapy the patient has had, which will often lead to the diagnosis.

Examination

Inspection will reveal the surgical scars and chest deformity which may result from surgery or the disease process. Remember to examine the trachea for deviation and to palpate the ribs for metastases. Percussion and auscultation should be used to detect the extent of the anatomical distortion following surgery.

Investigation

As in the case of most pulmonary problems, blood tests and radiology are useful investigations.

Key questions

1. What are the signs and causes of a pleural effusion?
2. What are the possible symptoms and signs of a bronchogenic carcinoma?
3. What signs are found on inspection and auscultation of a patient with mitral valve replacement?
4. Where would you listen for aortic and mitral valve murmurs, and what would you expect to hear?

7

Breast

Since breast cancer is a common condition (affecting one in 12 women in the UK), it appears commonly in surgical finals, in a patient with either primary cancer prior to surgery or (for longer cases) treated breast cancer. Patients with a fibroadenoma, cysts, nipple discharge or an abscess are also drafted into surgical finals.

HISTORY

A general history from breast patients should include age; menopausal status; age at menarche; age at menopause; number of pregnancies; hormone use (contraceptive pills, hormone replacement therapy); breast feeding; personal history of breast problems; and family history of breast disease. Ask whether family members have had breast cancer, and if so ask about other forms of cancer. Ask about smoking (associated with periductal inflammation) and gynaecological surgery (oophorectomy is protective against breast cancer).

If the patient admits to a change in the shape of one breast or a breast lump, ask when the lump was noticed; whether there have been any changes in the lump or the skin overlying it; whether there has been any nipple discharge (single duct/multiple ducts/blood-stained/colour?); whether there has been any breast pain/discomfort (breast cancers are usually painless); and whether any other lumps have been noted (for example in the axilla). In the case of patients who have breast cancer, ask about symptoms of possible metastatic disease such as bone pain, breathlessness, tiredness and anorexia.

EXAMINATION

Exposure/position

The patient should be unclothed from the waist upwards, and sitting on the edge of a couch or bed at the beginning of the examination.

Inspection

Look at the patient's breast and chest wall, first with the patient in the sitting position with hands on hips. Is there any visible abnormality or asymmetry of the breasts? Is there one breast or two? Ask the patient to reach above her head, and look for skin dimpling, peau d'orange (the skin looking like the skin of an orange), nipple retraction or any distortion. A cancer may be apparent first on inspection.

Remember to look for surgical scars (which may be quite difficult to spot if in the skin lines beneath the breast or in the axillary skin) and skin signs of radiotherapy (e.g. telangiectasis, breast distortion, skin which is shiny, thin or coarse).

Look for the encrusted, eczematous nipple of Paget's disease (which is unilateral, not itchy and does not usually occur in an atopic individual, unlike eczema).

Palpation

Ask the patient to lie flat on her back with one pillow and examine each breast systematically in turn. For examination of the left breast, the patient should place her left hand behind her head, and similarly for the right breast. Gently palpate the breast tissue, including the axillary tail of the breast, with flattened fingers to identify any lumps. If there is a lump, comment on its characteristics as follows:

- size – ideally measured with calipers
- shape – discrete lump(s) or diffuse swelling?
- position – which breast?
        – which quadrant of the breast?
        – inner or outer aspect?
        – position on the clock face
- fixation – tethering or fixation to the skin or underlying muscle

- consistency – hard/craggy/soft/tender/fluctuant?
- additional features – single or multiple?
  - axillary/cervical lymphadenopathy?
  - lumps in the contralateral breast?

To test for fixation to the chest wall, the patient should tense her chest wall muscles while you try to move the lump. If the lump is mobile when the patient is relaxed but fixed when the pectoralis major is tightened, then the tumour is tethered to the muscle.

Despite the inaccuracy of clinical examination in determining whether small axillary lymph nodes are involved with metastatic tumour, you still need to examine the regional lymph nodes. To examine for axillary lymph nodes, take the patient's left arm with yours, then using your right hand, examine the four walls of the axilla (medial, lateral, anterior, posterior) and its apex for palpable lymph nodes. Note where the nodes are palpable, whether there are a few scattered ('shotty') nodes (the sort you may well be able to feel in your own axilla), or large or matted nodes, and whether they are fixed to the surrounding structures. Whether or not you can feel any lymphadenopathy in the axilla, it is also mandatory to examine the infraclavicular, supraclavicular and cervical regions for lymphadenopathy, noting the presence of nodes as for the axilla.

Summary

Summarize the findings. For example, a summary of the case illustrated in Figure 7.1 might be 'A 60-year-old woman with a single, palpable, 2 cm, hard, non-tender lump in the 10 o'clock position of the upper outer quadrant of the right breast, 3 cm from the areolar margin. Not fixed to the deeper tissues but tethered to the skin. There are associated palpable matted 1 cm lymph nodes fixed to each other, and palpable in the medial wall of the axilla, though no supraclavicular or cervical lymphadenopathy.'

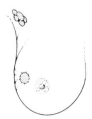

Fig. 7.1 Breast carcinoma

You may be asked if there is any other part of the patient you wish to examine: this is to remind you to examine the contralateral breast for a second cancer and the liver for metastatic disease. Examination of the abdomen for hepatomegaly is part of the follow-up clinical examination of a patient with breast cancer, and should be mentioned to the examiner.

INVESTIGATION

Key points

- Diagnosis of a breast lump is by triple assessment:
  - clinical
  - radiological
  - cytopathology

After the examination, the next task is to establish whether this lump is a cancer or not. Current guidelines dictate 'triple modality' diagnostic criteria for a clinically suspicious lump: clinically a cancer, a cancer mammographically and a cancer on fine needle aspiration cytology (or core biopsy) (see Fig. 7.2).

Mammography This is performed in two views on each breast: craniocaudal (up/down view) and oblique (showing the axillary tail of the breast, part of pectoralis major and the breast itself), and may be supplemented by magnification views. Mammography may demonstrate normal architecture (with breast tissue of variable density, usually most dense in young women); distorted architecture; masses or (micro) calcification. The two breasts are compared for differences in architecture. About 95% of breast cancers show up on mammography. (see Radiology chapter).

Breast ultrasound This is particularly useful in the under-35 age group, because mammography of dense breast tissue is difficult to interpret. Ultrasound scanning can be used to examine areas of lumpy breast, and may distinguish a common benign lump such as a fibroadenoma from a cancer by virtue of the outline of the lump and the acoustic shadow cast.

Fine needle aspiration cytology (FNAC) This involves inserting an 18-gauge (green) needle on a 10–20 ml syringe into the palpable area, and passing the needle to and fro through the

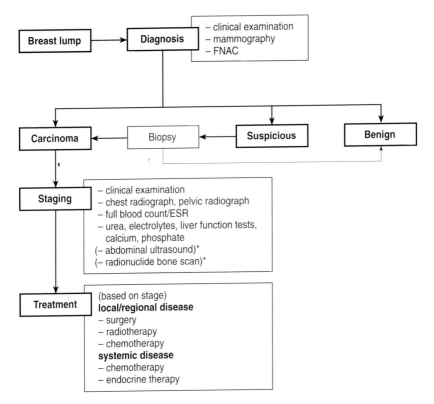

* for advanced disease

Fig. 7.2 Investigation of a breast lump

area 10+ times while gentle suction is applied using the syringe. The aspirate (which may be quite scanty) is then expressed onto glass slides, spread and either air-dried or fixed. A cytopathologist can subsequently examine the (stained) slides for cells, including breast cancer cells. In good hands (i.e. aspirator and cytopathologist) the diagnostic success rate is over 95%. FNAC can be performed either freehand (in the case of a palpable lump) or (for an impalpable breast lesion) using ultrasound or stereotactic mammography guidance.

Radiological tests These include a chest radiograph (for lung metastases or pleural effusion, liver ultrasound scan (reserved for advanced cancers, in which liver metastases are more likely); plain radiographs of symptomatic bony areas; and an isotope bone scan (for bone metastases).

Other investigations   These may include a full blood count (for anaemia, marrow infiltration, white count pre- and post-chemotherapy); erythrocyte sedimentation rate (may be raised in malignancy); levels of urea, electrolytes and creatinine (renal impairment may influence the choice and dosage of chemotherapy); and liver function tests (though a poor indicator of liver metastases).

MANAGEMENT

On the basis of the diagnostic and clinical tests, the patient can be 'staged' according to the TNM (Tumour Node Metastasis) system or as stage I, II, III, IV and the most suitable management of the individual patient can be decided. For patients with breast cancer, this may include surgery to the breast (lump or breast removal); surgery to the axilla (axillary node sampling or clearance); radiotherapy of the breast/chest wall and/or axillary tissues; endocrine therapy (e.g. tamoxifen, medroxyprogesterone); endocrine ablation (e.g. LHRH (luteinizing hormone releasing hormone) analogues, oophorectomy); and chemotherapy (bolus or infusional; before surgery, or postoperatively as adjuvant therapy; conventional or high dose). Which therapy to give to whom (and when) is best addressed by a multidisciplinary team including surgeon, chemotherapist, radiation oncologist, pathologist and nurse counsellor.

TYPICAL CASES

Single breast lump*

History

A single breast lump is a common breast problem in the final surgical exam. In women under 30 years of age, a single breast lump is most likely to be benign (benign breast tissue or, if discrete, a fibroadenoma – see Fig. 7.3), although it could be malignant. In the age range 30–45 years it is likely to be a cyst (see section below headed 'Multiple breast lumps') or carcinoma. Over 45 years of age, a single breast lump should be considered to be a breast cancer until proven otherwise (see Fig. 7.1).

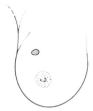

Fig. 7.3 Fibroadenoma

Examination

Follow the examination plan described above. If the patient turns out to have a single breast lump which you suspect may be a cancer, discuss the possible management with the examiner as outlined above.

In a young woman, normal breast tissue may give the impression of a discrete lump, which should fade away after her menses. A truly discrete lump, which is usually very mobile (hence its name 'breast mouse'), is likely to be a fibroadenoma and more than one may be present in the breast. Figure 7.3 shows a 24-year-old woman with a 1 cm firm, very mobile, smooth lump in the upper outer quadrant of the right breast (fibroadenoma).

Investigation

Clinical diagnosis should be backed up by mammography (in patients over 35 years of age), breast ultrasound and FNAC. The importance of a fibroadenoma lies in distinguishing it from more sinister breast lumps – once the diagnosis of a fibroadenoma has been established, most of these lumps do not need to be removed, and remain static in size for some years. However, if a clinician harbours residual doubts about a diagnosis, or if the patient strongly requests excision of a lump, then the lump should be removed (under local or general anaesthetic). If a cancer is diagnosed, the staging investigations outlined above are used to decide whether breast conservation is practicable. In general, for breast conservation the tumour should be 4 cm or less in size, without skin or chest wall involvement, and the breast should be large enough to allow excision of the tumour and a rim of breast tissue without unduly distorting the breast.

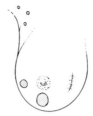

Fig. 7.4 Multiple breast lumps

Multiple breast lumps*

Multiple breast lumps in a patient in the exam are most likely to be breast cysts in a middle-aged woman. However, occasionally patients with benign lumpy breasts, multiple fibroadenomata or bilateral or multiple breast cancers may find their way into the exam.

History and examination

History-taking and examination should be as outlined above. Women with breast cysts have often experienced them before. They appear as lumps which are smooth and usually non-tender, often in both breasts. They may appear to be single or multiple and either small or quite large, and may even distort the size and shape of the breasts quite considerably. Bilateral breast examination should be followed by examination of the axillary, infraclavicular/supraclavicular and cervical nodes. Figure 7.4 shows a 45-year-old woman with two 2–3 cm lumps in the 6 o'clock and 9 o'clock positions of the right breast. The lumps are smooth in outline, non-tender and mobile. There is also a surgical scar in the 3 o'clock position, and 'shotty' lymph nodes in the axilla. This patient had cysts and had previously had a breast biopsy.

Investigation

Mammography (or preferably breast ultrasound in a patient under 35 years of age) will reveal the well circumscribed outline of a cyst, and should be used to help exclude any other impalpable breast pathology. Aspiration with a needle and syringe will confirm the diagnosis, and treat the cysts. The colour of the cystic fluid which may be clear, opalescent, or green through to almost black) and its volume (usually 5–20 ml, but occasionally up to 100 ml) are of

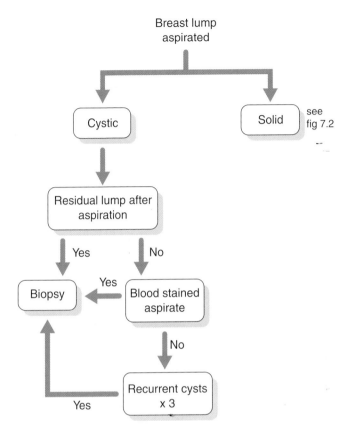

Fig. 7.5 Indications for biopsy of breast cyst

little consequence. However, a bloody aspirate, a residual mass after aspiration or cysts which recur a third time after two aspirations 3 weeks apart, may indicate an underlying cancer and such areas should be excised (Fig. 7.5). Patients with multiple cysts may decide to live with their cysts, asking for only particularly prominent lumps to be aspirated.

Post-mastectomy patient*

History

In addition to the basic breast history already outlined, patients who have undergone treatment for breast cancer may be asked what surgery they have had (particularly to the breast, axilla and abdomen); whether they have had radiation therapy (to the breast or chest wall alone or to the axilla also) and/or chemotherapy (before or after surgery, or both); and what medications they have had previously and are now taking, and for how long.

Examination

Inspect the chest and compare the two sides for scars: a mastectomy scar is usually transverse, sometimes angling up into the axilla. Most mastectomy operations now leave the pectoralis major muscle in place (i.e. modified radical or Patey mastectomy) rather than involving radical mastectomy (with removal of pectoralis major). Look for the signs of radiotherapy: vascular telangiectasia of the skin in the field of irradiation, which may include the infra- or supraclavicular regions in addition to the chest wall. Diffuse skin-thickening may also occur after radiotherapy, or the skin may appear thin, shiny and atrophic.

As a consequence of axillary node clearance and/or axillary radiotherapy or axillary nodal disease, some patients develop upper limb oedema which appears as mild to severe swelling of the hand, forearm and/or upper arm. Figure 7.6 shows a mastectomy scar and a lymphoedematous arm following modified radical mastectomy and axillary node clearance.

Remember to inspect the other breast (if present) for features of breast disease.

Palpation over the treated post-mastectomy chest wall should include feeling for any skin nodules (tumour metastases or buried sutures?) and up into the axilla for nodes or masses. The supraclavicular, infraclavicular and cervical nodes should also be palpated.

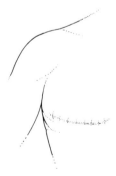

Fig. 7.6 Post-mastectomy patient

Investigations

Investigations performed routinely in post-mastectomy patients include annual mammography of the contralateral breast, to detect a second primary breast cancer (detected in 1–3% of patients per annum).

Breast conservation patient[†]

History

Breast conservation is the term used to describe patients who have had a breast cancer removed (lumpectomy) but in whom the remainder of the breast has been conserved (see Fig. 7.7). So, after asking the general breast history questions, you will need to ask patients who have undergone breast conservation treatment what surgery they have had to the breast (e.g. was the lumpectomy successful at the first excision?); axilla (were the lymph nodes sampled or cleared from the axilla?) and abdomen (was oophorectomy performed?). Many breast conservation patients have adjuvant radiotherapy of the residual breast (and axilla unless the nodes have been cleared) in case of microscopic residual disease, and adjuvant endocrine therapy (such as tamoxifen) or chemotherapy (particularly for premenopausal women with node involvement): you will need to ask about these aspects of the patient's treatment.

Examination

Inspect and compare the two breasts in terms of general size, shape and contour. Look for scars on the breast (from lumpectomy) and in the axilla (from node excision). After breast conservation there may be distortion of the appearance of the breast. There may also

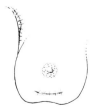

Fig. 7.7 Breast conservation patient

be signs of radiotherapy, particularly diffuse skin thickening. Remember to inspect both breasts thoroughly. Figure 7.7 shows a lumpectomy scar (with some breast distortion) and an axillary scar (from an axillary node procedure). Look also for regional nodes (supraclavicular) and skin changes due to radiotherapy.

Palpation over the treated breast should include the lumpectomy site (where there may be palpable scar tissue), the residual breast tissue (for further lumps) and then the axilla and the supraclavicular, infraclavicular and cervical nodes. Do not forget to examine the untreated breast.

Annual mammography of the treated breast and the contralateral side should be carried out, to detect recurrent disease or a second primary breast cancer. Long-term survival is no worse after lumpectomy than after mastectomy.

Gynaecomastia[†]

History

Gynaecomastia usually has one of three causes: physiological (in young men); induced by drugs (particularly cimetidine, or cardiac drugs including digoxin and spironolactone); or a systemic hormonal upset (particularly liver disease, hormonal therapy for prostate cancer, or testicular or pituitary tumours). Therefore the history should include the patient's age and the timing of onset and duration of the swollen breast tissue. Is the gynaecomastia unilateral or bilateral? Is it tender or embarrassing? Ask about alcohol intake and drug history (with particular regard to cardiac or prostate cancer therapy), and whether the patient has had prostate surgery or noted a lump in the testicle.

Examination

Examination of the male breast should be performed as for the female breast: often, simple exposure of the torso with the patient sitting and then inspection will suggest the diagnosis of gynaecomastia. If the underlying cause of the gynaecomastia is hepatic, some of the many signs of liver disease may be visible. You are unlikely to be asked to examine a man with breast cancer, but remember that male breast cancer does exist. It usually presents in elderly men at a locally advanced stage (including skin infiltration and often nodal disease too).

Before palpation of the breast tissue, ask whether it is tender. Usually gynaecomastia is palpable as a firm retroareolar mass, although it may be to one side of the breast area. Palpate for axillary and cervical lymphadenopathy, and remember to check the contralateral side.

The examination of a man with gynaecomastia should include the testes, since gynaecomastia is a possible presentation of testicular cancer. You should mention this in the exam, but you are unlikely to be asked to perform testicular examination on such a patient.

Investigation

The investigation of gynaecomastia should be aimed at determining the nature of the lump (to exclude carcinoma) and excluding serious pathology elsewhere. Fine needle aspiration cytology can be used to confirm the diagnosis.

Ultrasound scanning of a testicular lump, radiological views of the pituitary fossa and/or serum prolactin level may all be suggested as suitable investigations. Investigations for liver disease (see Ch. 8) may be appropriate in a patient with other signs of hepatic disease.

Treatment

The two main methods of treatment are discontinuation of a medication reponsible for the gynaecomastia (which should result in a reduction of the swelling) and surgical excision of the offending tissue (if the patient wishes).

Breast cancer metastasis[§]

Breast cancer may commonly metastasize, usually to bones, liver, lungs, pleurae, peritoneal cavity, brain or subcutaneous tissues. A patient with metastatic breast cancer may be used as a long case in surgical finals, or as a short case for the detection of ascites, a palpable liver or a pleural effusion.

Nipple discharge[§]

Nipple discharge is a common symptom, usually physiological. You need to ask whether the discharge is from one nipple or both; whether it is from only one duct on the nipple; and what colour it is (clear (physiological), milky due to galactorrhoea, greenish or cheesy due to duct ectasia, or brown or blood-stained due to a duct papilloma or carcinoma).

The detection of blood in the discharge requires you to test for blood with a dipstick unless frank red blood is being emitted from the nipple. Clearly, there will be concern about a blood-stained discharge from a single duct, which may signify an underlying carcinoma. Other investigations, including mammography, should aim to exclude a cancer.

Nipple eczema[§]

Nipples which appear to be eczematous may be just that, but beware of Paget's disease of the nipple (breast carcinoma cells in the nipple skin), which can have an identical appearance. Thus if a woman who is middle-aged or older, and has no skin problems elsewhere, presents with nipple eczema, you will need to exclude Paget's disease and an underlying carcinoma.

Breast abscess[§]

A breast abscess is usually so painful that the woman concerned is unlikely to consent to appearing in an exam. Breast abscesses occur in breastfeeding mothers and in smokers. You should look for the features of inflammation (hot, red, tender, swollen, loss of function). Resolution may be achieved by using antibiotics, by aspiration of the pus under antibiotic cover, or by open drainage. Be aware that an inflammatory carcinoma of the breast may present with all the appearances of an abscess.

Skin lesions[§]

Skin lesions (e.g. sebaceous cyst, papilloma, lipoma) may occur on the breast and adjacent chest wall.

Key questions

1. What questions would you ask a patient with breast symptoms?
2. How do you describe a breast cancer after clinical examination?
3. How would you diagnose a breast cancer?
4. What are the clinical features of a breast cancer on examination?
5. Where does breast cancer metastasize to? *Bones, Brain, Liver, Lung, Peritoneal cavy, Pleure,*
6. What are the common diagnoses of a breast lump in a 30-year-old woman, a 40-year-old woman and a 70-year-old woman? *↳Fibroaden →cysts →Ca.*
7. What features of previous breast cancer treatment might you see on the chest wall? *↳ Scars (lumpecty, mastecy) → Skin changes → Irradiation. →*

8

Abdomen

Abdominal examination forms one of the key parts of surgical finals. Students often worry about where to start in a short case when asked to 'examine the gastrointestinal system' which (confusingly) means start with the hands, examine the head and neck, look in the mouth and examine the chest wall *before* you approach the abdomen. On the other hand, when an examiner asks you to 'examine the abdomen' in surgical circles, he or she means exactly that!

Key points

- The history (70%), examination (20%) and investigations (10%) contribute to the diagnosis of abdominal disorders

HISTORY

If you have a patient with an abdominal problem for your long case, it is important that in your systematic enquiry you remember to ask all the questions relevant to gastrointestinal disease. It may be useful to begin with general questions, covering appetite; weight loss or gain (which may be in terms of pounds, kilograms or a change in size of clothing or belt); nausea; pallor; or jaundice. Then move from one end of the gastrointestinal tract to the other.

Ask about ulcers or discomfort in the mouth; tooth or denture problems; taste and salivary gland swelling. Enquire about swallowing and dysphagia in relation to solids, liquids and (in extreme circumstances) saliva. If vomiting is a symptom, when does the vomiting occur – immediately after eating, or 1 hour or more later?

Is food readily recognizable (regurgitated), partly digested or fully digested? Is indigestion, heartburn or waterbrash (fluid regurgitating to the back of the throat) a symptom, and if so when does it occur?

Does the patient experience abdominal pain, and if so, what are its features?

- When does it occur?
- Where does it occur?
- Can the pain be described (sharp/dull/burning)?
- How often does the pain occur?
- Where does the pain radiate to?
- What are the aggravating features?
- What are the relieving features?
- What are the associated features?

Some conditions have characteristic patterns of pain (e.g. colicky central abdominal pain, moving to become constant right iliac fossa pain in appendicitis). Is there any abdominal bloating or distension? Is this episodic?

Has there been any change in bowel habit, or any constipation or diarrhoea? If so, what are the consistency, colour, smell and features of the stool? (Does it float, or flush easily?) Has the patient passed any mucus, pus or blood per anum? If blood has been noted, was it red or dark; clots or liquid; mixed with the stool or on the toilet paper; on one occasion or many? Is there pain on defaecation or any faecal or urinary incontinence? Have there been problems with abscesses or fistulae in the anal area? Is there any perianal itch?

Family history may be of particular relevance in the case of colorectal cancer (which may also be associated with breast or ovarian cancer: remember to ask), inflammatory bowel disease and rare conditions such as familial adenomatous polyposis, Peutz–Jehgers syndrome or hereditary haemorrhagic telangiectasia. Similarly, the smoking, alcohol and drug history may point to the diagnosis. The history of how the condition has been treated in the past, is currently under treatment, hospital admissions and operations will also yield pointers as to the diagnosis.

Thus, by the time you actually examine a patient with an abdominal condition in a long case, you will probably know, or at least have a very good idea about, the diagnosis and what you are likely to find. In a short case, if you are not allowed to ask questions, you may still get a lot of clues by using your powers of observation as you approach the patient.

EXAMINATION

Remember that, in a short case, the examiner will be watching to see how you conduct an examination of the patient, and this is perhaps even more important than what you find. Approach the patient so as to be at his or her right-hand side. Then introduce yourself – this is a good way to start, as it breaks the ice.

Exposure/position

Position the patient (flat on his or her back, head resting on one pillow, hands by sides, legs uncrossed) so as to be comfortable and relaxed, with adequate exposure from nipples to groin (it used to be nipples to knees). Even if you are asked to 'examine the abdomen', you may get clues as you expose and position the patient by looking at the face (for spider naevi, telangiectasia or perioral pigmented spots), hands (for clubbing, palmar erythema, Dupuytren's contracture) or chest (for a missing breast, gynaecomastia). Be prepared to mention these features when you describe what you can see on inspection.

Inspection

Inspection can give you many clues (e.g. scars, stomata, skin changes, large masses) as to what you may find during subsequent examination of the patient. Watch for movement on respiration, visible peristalsis, and abdominal asymmetry. The secret is to show that you are looking but not bore the examiner by the length of time that you take.

Ensure that you are seen to look for not just obvious scars (Fig. 8.1), but also scars on the left flank (left nephrectomy, left thoracic approach, iliac crest bone excision), in the groin (from vascular procedures or hernias, and sometimes hidden by hair or fat), at the umbilicus and even on the chest wall (sternotomy). Not all scars are big and some heal remarkably well, particularly laparoscopic wounds and incisions in the skin lines or groin creases.

Look for obvious skin changes (e.g. distended veins, skin lesions, bruising, erythema ab igne), masses, stomata (which may be hidden by the stoma bag) and fistulae. If there is a stoma (Fig. 8.2) ask yourself: Where is it in the abdomen? Does it protrude from or is it flush with the abdominal surface? What is it producing (solids, liquid stool

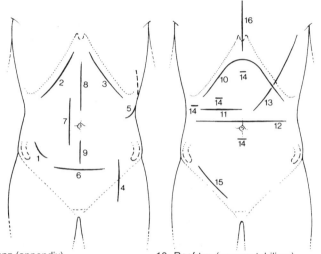

Key

1. Lanz (appendix)
2. Kocher's (hepatobiliary)
3. Left subcostal (spleen)
4. Vascular
5. Nephrectomy (extraperitoneal)
6. Pfannensteil (gynaecology or caesarean section)
7. Paramedian
8. Upper midline
9. Lower midline

10. Roof-top (pancreatobiliary)
11. Transverse (gallbladder, colectomy)
12. Transverse (abdominal aortic aneurysm, colonic surgery)
13. Thoracoabdominal (extending over left thorax: gastro-oesophageal surgery)
14. Laparoscopic port sites
15. Inguinal hernia
16. Sternotomy

Fig. 8.1 Abdominal scars

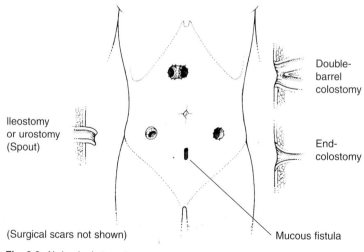

Double-barrel colostomy

Ileostomy or urostomy (Spout)

End-colostomy

(Surgical scars not shown)

Mucous fistula

Fig. 8.2 Abdominal stomata

or urine)? Is there one opening or two? Remember that a colostomy is usually (but not exclusively) in the LIF (left iliac fossa), should lie flush with the skin and when mature produces a formed stool. An ileostomy should protrude as a 2–3 cm spout to protect the surrounding skin, is often located in the RIF (right iliac fossa), and produces liquid stool, sometimes in considerable amounts. Either a colostomy or an ileostomy can be an end-stoma or a loop of bowel brought to the surface as a loop-stoma (or double-barrel stoma). To add to the potential confusion, end-stomata and loop-stomata produce bowel content whereas a mucous fistula (usually an end of sigmoid colon) does not, being one end of a defunctioned length of bowel. A urostomy may look similar to the spout of an ileostomy, but involves an isolated length of ileum into which the ureters have been plumbed, which acts as a conduit for urine. A urostomy produces urine, recognizable by its colour, though often a little cloudy due to the ileal mucus production.

The complications of an abdominal stoma include retraction, prolapse, stenosis, parastomal hernia and dehydration/electrolyte imbalance.

Abdominal masses are sometimes apparent just by observation of a quietly breathing patient. Asking the patient to lift his or her head off the pillow and/or asking for a 'big cough' to make a hernia protrude (particularly an incisional hernia secondary to previous surgery) will be obvious even to your examiner. Even so, point out the visible abnormality to your examiner and state what you have observed on inspection, then move on to palpation.

Palpation

Ask the patient's permission to examine (palpate) his or her abdomen, and before you start ensure that both of you are in a comfortable position. Kneeling beside the bed at the patient's right-hand side (not sitting on the bed) is one ideal position in the eyes of some examiners. Before you touch the patient ask 'Are you sore anywhere?', and if so ask him or her to point out the tender areas. Leave touching any painful areas until last. Watch the patient's face (to see if you are causing discomfort) and gently palpate, rotating between the four quadrants of the abdomen. Follow this with deeper (but still gentle) palpation. By now you should have identified and delineated any obvious masses. If you feel a mass, make sure that you define its extent (this may be difficult for a mass arising from the pelvis, in which case you should say so). What is the size of the mass? Is it possible to indent the mass (faeces will indent)? Can you ballott the mass? Is it expansile (i.e. an aneurysm)?

Palpation for specific features

The liver To feel for the edge of the liver, start in the right iliac fossa and palpate towards the right costal margin, using the tips of your fingers gently applied to the abdominal wall. The edge of the liver, if palpable, will move inferiorly with each deep inspiration, and will meet your fingers. Be careful to ensure that if you feel a mass you cannot insinuate your fingers between this and the costal margin – if this is possible it is not the liver you are feeling! You can then define the lower border of the liver and state how far (in cm) it lies below the costal margin. You cannot state that the liver is enlarged until you have defined (by percussion) its upper border (normally in the midclavicular line of the fourth intercostal space). If in doubt as to the position of the lower border of the liver, listen with your stethoscope over the presumed liver edge and use your index finger to gently scratch the skin along a line perpendicular to the presumed edge and extending across it (from the skin overlying the liver to that over the rest of the abdomen). There is a change in the quality and pitch of the sound heard as you pass from solid (liver) to hollow organ (intestines). Having felt a liver edge, state whether the liver is tender or not. Is the liver smooth (usually benign) or craggy (often neoplastic); soft or firm; pulsatile (suggesting tricuspid regurgitation) or hard (tumour)? As you examine, sneak a look for other general signs which might lead you to likely causes of hepatomegaly (see below).

Key points

- Start in (R) iliac fossa and palpate towards (R)costal margin
- Feel whole length of liver border
- Comment on tenderness and consistency of liver

The spleen Again start in the right iliac fossa (not the left iliac fossa or you may miss a large spleen), palpating as for a liver edge but this time towards the left costal margin. If you cannot feel the spleen, roll the patient towards you (to lie on their right side) and feel under the left costal margin on deep inspiration. Comment on whether it is possible to palpate 'above' the spleen (i.e. between the spleen and the costal margin): this should not be possible in the case of the spleen, but should be possible in the case of an enlarged left kidney. The spleen typically has a palpable notch which may distinguish it from other masses.

Key points

- Start in (R) iliac fossa feeling towards (L) costal margin
- Consider rotation of the patient if difficult to feel

The kidneys   Using bimanual palpation on inspiration, try to palpate each kidney in turn. Place the flat of one hand behind the patient, under the loin, and the other hand on the upper quadrant of the same side. On deep inspiration, a normal kidney may just be palpable in a thin person (particularly on the right-hand side, where it lies a little lower than on the left), descending to meet your anterior hand. You may also try to ballott the kidney with a sharp push from the posterior hand, pressing the kidney towards your other (anterior) hand. Even large kidneys (which are usually polycystic if really big) should not stop you from 'getting above' the kidney under the rib-cage, which should not be possible in the case of the liver or spleen, If you percuss over an enlarged kidney the note is often resonant as there will be overlying bowel gas – another means of determining if the mass you are feeling is really a kidney.

A word of caution: a transplanted kidney is usually placed in the right iliac fossa (where the renal artery and vein can be readily connected to the iliac vessels, and the ureter to the bladder). It is readily palpable, as a smooth subcutaneous mass beneath a scar very like a long appendectomy scar – a sneaky trick putting it there, but if you know it's a possibility, forewarned is forearmed.

Key points

- Kidneys are ballottable
- You should be able to get your hand above the (L) kidney
- Percussion over either kidney is generally resonant

Aortic aneurysm   An abdominal aortic aneurysm (AAA) can be missed unless you remember to palpate specifically for an expansile mass adjacent to the umbilicus. Place your index fingers on either side of the line of the aorta, gently pressing to feel the sensation of the fingers being pushed apart. It is difficult to comment on the size of an abdominal aortic aneurysm without ultrasound scanning, but in a thin person an aneurysm may be readily palpable.

Key points

- An abdominal aortic aneurysm is truly expansile
- This will differentiate if from transmitted pulsation via an overlying mass

Percussion

Percuss all four quadrants of the abdomen. Don't press too hard when trying to percuss, and make sure your fingernails are not so long as to leave your hand sore. Percuss the margins of any masses you have already identified. Is the mass tympanic or solid? Percuss the upper and lower borders of the liver and spleen, and the upper border of the bladder or uterus (occasionally a pregnant woman finds her way into finals).

Shifting dullness due to ascites is often easier to demonstrate by percussion than by demonstrating a fluid thrill: successive percussion of your finger placed over the patient's flank, parallel to the spine, will delineate the fluid/air interface. Keep your finger over a place that has been dull to percussion as the patient rolls onto his or her side, then percuss again – if the dull note has become resonant, shifting dullness has been demonstrated.

Auscultation

Remember to listen for bowel sounds (frequency, pitch, isolated/runs) over the abdomen, and if appropriate over any hernia. Runs of frequent, high-pitched bowel sounds can be heard when the bowel is obstructed. If the bowel sounds are scanty or absent (make sure you listen for long enough), ileus or peritonitis is indicated.

Remember to listen for a hepatic bruit (suggesting hepatoma). If necessary, auscultate for the edge of the liver using the 'scratch' test described above. With the patient sitting, listen in the renal angle for a renal artery bruit posteriorly, and listen for femoral artery bruits in the groin.

To seek a succussion splash (if you suspect gastric outflow obstruction), gently shake the supine patient from side to side then hold him or her still and listen. (You can sometimes hear your own succussion splash if you move around actively after a meal.)

Further examination

Finally, state that you would normally proceed to perform a digital rectal examination of every patient. It is usually said that there can be only two reasons for not doing so: either the patient has no anus (e.g. following abdominoperineal excision of the rectum) or you have no fingers. In an exam there is a third reason – the fact that it is an exam, and patients would not participate if they thought they would have to undergo multiple rectal examinations. Vaginal examination should also be mentioned if this would be appropriate, but similarly you are not likely to be expected to perform this in the exam.

You must not forget that a basic abdominal examination should include testing a urine sample (for protein, blood, and glucose as a minimum) and testing stool for faecal occult blood. You may be provided with a patient's urine sample to test in the exam.

TYPICAL CASES

Abdominal mass*

Key points

- The patient's age and history and the position of an abdominal mass suggests the likely diagnosis
- This should be confirmed by appropriate investigation

An abdominal mass is amongst the most common of problems to be presented to you in the surgical exams. Most abdominal masses will be intra-abdominal, although masses may also indicate abdominal wall lesions such as a lipoma, rectus muscle haematoma or a rare abdominal wall tumour. A lump within the abdominal wall is still palpable when the abdominal wall is tensed (e.g. when the patient lifts their head off the pillow), but an intra-abdominal mass is not.

History

Remember to ask about gastrointestinal symptoms, urinary symptoms and gynaecological symptoms. The past medical history and, particularly, a history of surgical operations can be most helpful in suggesting the diagnosis.

Examination

Follow the scheme of exposure/positioning, inspection, palpation, percussion, auscultation – bearing in mind the anatomical structures present in each area and the possible causes of a palpable mass in each region. An abdominal mass is typically inflammatory or neoplastic. Figure 8.3 summarizes the possible locations and

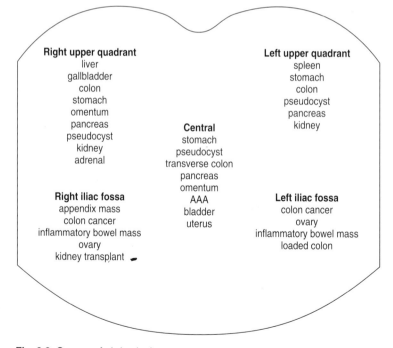

Fig. 8.3 Causes of abdominal masses

causes of abdominal masses. Remember that intra-abdominal lymph nodes and rare conditions such as a mesenteric cyst (a smooth swelling which is very mobile) may occur in any region of the abdomen. Your examiners will be more interested in your approach to the patient and their problem than necessarily the correct diagnosis.

Investigation

Decide what investigations you need to define the pathology; start with the least invasive and progress to the more complex investigations. Always include basic biochemistry (urea, electrolytes, liver function tests, creatinine) and haematology (haemoglobin, white cell count, platelets, ESR). Test the urine (for glucose, blood, protein and bilirubin particularly), test for pregnancy in women of child-bearing age, and test for faecal occult blood.

Radiology   Select appropriate investigations from plain abdominal films; abdominal ultrasound scanning (needs a fasting patient, to ensure full gallbladder and reduced bowel gas); pelvic ultrasound (needs a full bladder to act as an acoustic window into the pelvis); intravenous urogram (IVU); and computed tomography (CT) scan (which may be performed with intravenous and/or oral contrast to delineate specific structures). For upper gastrointestinal problems, use a barium or water-soluble contrast as a swallow/meal/follow-through/small bowel enema. For lower gastrointestinal problems, give a contrast enema per anum (either single-contrast, such as barium, or double-contrast, such as barium and air).

Special tests   Upper gastrointestinal endoscopy can be used to examine the oesophagus, stomach and duodenum (usually to the second part). It is ideally performed on a fasting patient (so that the stomach is empty), with local anaesthetic throat spray and/or intravenous sedation if required. Rigid proctoscopy and rigid sigmoidoscopy are somewhat misnamed, since the proctoscope provides adequate examination of the anal canal but not the proctum (rectum) and the sigmoidoscope provides adequate examination of the rectum (perhaps as high as the rectosigmoid junction), but not of the sigmoid colon. The sigmoid colon and rectum can be examined by flexible sigmoidoscopy. The complete large bowel to the ileocaecal valve (and sometimes the terminal ileum too) can be examined by colonoscopy, which is often performed with intravenous sedation.

Jaundice*

- Jaundice is usually post-hepatic in surgical finals
- Ultrasound is the single most useful investigation in
  determining if this is the case

Icteric patients are surprisingly common on surgical wards, and in a surgical context their jaundice usually has a post-hepatic cause. Prehepatic and hepatic jaundice are usually medical conditions, but should form part of your differential diagnosis in all jaundiced patients. Causes of jaundice to remember include:

- Prehepatic
  - transfusion reactions
  - haemolysis secondary to sepsis or haematological disease
- Hepatic
  - hepatitis (e.g. viral hepatitis A,B,C)
  - cirrhosis
  - drugs
- Post-hepatic
  - biliary obstruction due to gallstones
  - primary cancer (pancreas, cholangiocarcinoma, ampullary carcinoma)
  - metastatic carcinoma of the liver
  - secondary carcinoma (e.g. of portal nodes)
  - sclerosing cholangitis. ⟶ in UC rctcln
  - benign biliary structures.
    Strictures

History

Remember to ask about fever, itch, bruising, dark urine, pale stools and other bowel symptoms (including those of inflammatory bowel disease). Ask about the timing of the onset of the jaundice, and whether it is progressive or intermittent and/or associated with abdominal or back pain. Patients with viral hepatitis often give a history of prodromal symptoms occurring prior to their becoming frankly icteric. A history of travel abroad, blood transfusion, infectious contacts, tattoos, relevant occupation, alcohol or drugs (whether prescribed or not) or a family history (e.g. haemolytic) may lead you to a diagnosis.

Examination

With the patient lying comfortably, with one pillow and exposed from nipple to groin, inspect for the depth of jaundice; associated scratch marks (due to pruritus); pallor; bruising; nutritional state; and stigmata of chronic liver disease. These stigmata include spider naevi, palmar erythema, Dupuytren's contracture, bruising, flapping tremor, cerebral impairment, testicular atrophy, gynaecomastia, sparse body hair, peripheral oedema and caput medusae (a lot to spot at one glance!).

Palpate for lymphadenopathy in the neck, and for hepatomegaly, splenomegaly and testicular atrophy. Courvoisier's law is a common topic in surgical finals. In essence, it states that if the gallbladder is palpable in a jaundiced patient, then the jaundice is not likely to be due to gallstones. This law is not absolute. It relies on the finding that gallbladders containing stones are usually small and shrunken (and so impalpable), whereas gallbladder (and bile duct) distension may result from common bile duct obstruction, caused by, for example, a pancreatic carcinoma (hence the gallbladder is palpable where the ninth costal cartilage meets the costal margin).

Percuss for ascites (shifting dullness) and auscultate for a hepatic bruit.

An examination is theoretically incomplete without a rectal examination (for palpable tumour and occult or obvious blood) and urine testing. Testing the urine can enable you to distinguish between haemolytic jaundice (no bilirubin in the urine) and obstructive jaundice (water-soluble conjugated bilirubin in the urine, but no urobilinogen, due to interruption of the enterohepatic circulation).

Investigation

Investigations are summarized in Figure 8.4.

Urine test   Test for bilirubin and urobilinogen.

Basic haematology   Basic haematology, including coagulation and blood biochemistry should be performed to detect anaemia, raised white cell count (in cholangitis), and raised platelet count (in splenic infarction due to splenic vein obstruction). Look at the levels of urea and electrolytes (beware of renal failure with jaundice, which is a lethal combination). Serum sodium may be low in cirrhosis.

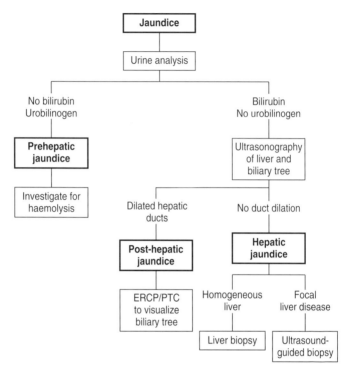

Fig. 8.4 Investigations for jaundice.

Liver function tests Alkaline phosphatase and bilirubin levels are raised disproportionately compared with those of ALT (alanine aminotransferase) and GGT (gamma-glutamyl transferase) in obstructive jaundice. ALT levels are particularly high in hepatic forms of jaundice, but with prolonged jaundice the distinction becomes less clear. Albumin levels can be low in chronic liver disease (<30 g/l – severe; <20 g/l – bad news). Clotting may be abnormal, reflecting poor synthetic function, and will need correction prior to ERCP (see below) or surgery using vitamin K or, in emergency, blood products.

Radiology Ultrasound scanning is useful for investigating gallstones; liver size and texture; hepatic lesions > 1 cm in size; dilated bile ducts (>10 mm in the case of the common bile duct); ascites; and splenomegaly. However, its usefulness is severely limited by obesity and by gaseous distension of the bowel (hence patients fast prior to scanning). A CT scan may provide the same information: it is less useful for investigating gallstones, but may be better for visualizing the pancreas, smaller hepatic lesions, portal anatomy and blood flow (on dynamic scan).

Special tests   Endoscopic retrograde cholangiopancreatography (ERCP), performed with a side-viewing endoscope, is ideal for examining the ampulla, pancreatic duct and biliary tree. Percutaneous transhepatic cholangiography (PTC) is useful if the biliary tree is dilated or if ERCP is not possible (either not available or due to a technical failure, e.g. because of a previous Polya gastrectomy). Liver biopsy and/or laparoscopy, with or without laparoscopic ultrasound scanning, may also contribute to the diagnosis. Note the advent of novel non-invasive imaging techniques, such as endoscopic ultrasound and magnetic resonance cholangiography, which may surpass ERCP and PTC as ways of imaging the biliary tree.

Management

In addition to being asked about the diagnostic pathway in icteric patients, you may be asked about the problems which occur when such patients are operated upon. These problems may be related to haemostasis; fluid and electrolyte balance and renal failure; and/or malnutrition and immunosuppression, leading to poor wound healing and increased risk of infection.

Ascites*

Key points

- Shifting dullness on clinical examination, confirmed by ultrasound

The causes of ascites in patients likely to appear in surgical finals include cirrhosis (patients may also show signs of portal hypertension, such as splenomegaly or prominent abdominal wall veins); malignancy (particularly gastrointestinal, ovarian or breast cancers); pancreatic ascites (secondary to pancreatitis with a high amylase level in the fluid); thrombosis of the portal vein following pancreatitis (may also lead to portal hypertension); hypoalbuminaemia (e.g. due to malnutrition, cirrhosis, cachexia in cancer); or obstruction/occlusion of the inferior vena cava or hepatic veins (known as Budd–Chiari syndrome in the latter case). Ascites may also be associated with pleural effusions or peripheral oedema.

History

Remember that the causes of abdominal distension can be summarized as the five 'Fs': flatus, fluid (ascites), faeces, fetus and fat. When exploring the patient's history, include questions on conditions which predispose to ascites such as malignancy, alcoholic cirrhosis, pancreatitis and cardiac failure.

Examination

With the patient adequately exposed and in the correct position, inspect for signs of chronic liver disease (in addition to ascites), including: palmar erythema; Dupuytren's contracture; spider naevi; flapping tremor; testicular atrophy; gynaecomastia; peripheral oedema; hepatosplenomegaly; caput medusae.

Test for shifting dullness (diagnostic of ascites) by percussion as outlined above. Confirmation of ascites can be obtained by looking for a fluid thrill – this requires an additional hand, and it is customary to ask the examiner for the use of his or her hand.

Investigation

Serum albumin, sodium and potassium levels are of particular importance.

Ultrasound scanning will demonstrate the ascitic fluid.

A diagnostic tap of the ascites (using an 18-gauge needle/ syringe into the right or left iliac fossa) can be used for the protein content, amylase level, cytology and bacteriology of the ascitic fluid.

Upper gastrointestinal endoscopy should be considered in patients with portal hypertension, to detect the presence of oesophageal varices.

Hepatomegaly*

Key points

- Neoplastic, cardiac and infective causes
- Blood and radiological diagnosis

The three most common causes of *apparent* hepatomegaly are: a normal but palpable lower border of the liver (hence the importance of percussion to identify the upper border); cardiac failure; and metastatic disease involving the liver.

History

Remember the cardiac, neoplastic (primary or metastatic) and infective causes of hepatomegaly.

Examination

Inspect for signs of generalized liver disease, malignancy, and cardiac failure.

Remember to define both the upper border of the liver (by percussion, in the fourth intercostal space in the midclavicular line) and the lower border (by palpation, percussion and/or the 'scratch' test). Ask yourself whether the edge of the liver is smooth/irregular, firm/soft, tender (e.g. in hepatitis, congestive cardiac failure) or pulsatile (e.g. with tricuspid regurgitation), and whether there is an audible bruit (e.g. with hepatoma). Examine for splenomegaly (see below).

Investigation

To supplement the routine haematological and biochemical investigations, the blood should be tested for AFP (alpha feto-protein, suggesting hepatoma) and CEA (carcinoembryonic antigen, suggesting colonic liver metastases).

An ultrasound scan, CAT (computerized axial tomography) scan, and, if required, liver biopsy and laparoscopy should be used to establish the diagnosis.

Dysphagia*

Key points

- Usually due to a disorder within the wall of the oesophagus (carcinoma or peptic stricture)
- Determine the severity of dysphagia and over what time-scale it has been present
- Upper endoscopy is the key to identifying surgical causes of dysphagia

Patients with dysphagia make a good long case. They are often elderly, and may have other disease states in addition to that causing the dysphagia. You must remember that dysphagia is always assumed to be due to a significant pathology – there may be: oral/pharyngeal causes (unlikely to appear in surgical finals) or oesophageal causes, which may be intralumenal, mural (e.g. carcinoma, benign stricture, scleroderma), extramural (e.g. goitre, nodes, lung cancer) or neurological/functional.

History

It is essential, first to grade dysphagia and, second, to determine whether it is progressive – if so, over what time-scale. Find out if the patient can swallow solids, semi-solids, liquids or has trouble with their own saliva (absolute dysphagia). Is this constant and progressive (often a tumour), constant but static (often a benign stricture) or intermittent (functional causes)? It is important to ask about weight loss, regurgitation and aspiration. If the patient is not sure about weight loss ask about how well (or not) their clothes fit.

The history should also include a full gastrointestinal enquiry. Remember to ask about medications (particularly NSAIDs (non-steroidal anti-inflammatory drugs), drugs for the treatment of ulcers or reflux, and iron).

Examination

On inspection, is the general impression of a well-nourished individual or is the patient cachectic, pale or jaundiced? Are there any signs of systemic disease, including rare conditions such as scleroderma?

Include in the examination the hands (for signs of e.g. loss of muscle mass, anaemia, scleroderma), then the head and neck (for systemic signs of malignant disease, particularly lymphadenopathy). Examine the chest, particularly for signs of lobar consolidation (due to aspiration) and for pleural effusion (secondary to consolidation or malignancy). Examine the abdomen for an upper abdominal mass (carcinoma of the gastro-oesophageal junction commonly presents with dysphagia) and for hepatomegaly (e.g. due to malignant disease).

Investigation

Investigations should include a full blood count, to detect anaemia in particular (e.g. due to oesophagitis or carcinoma of the upper gastrointestinal tract, or associated with an oesophageal web). Blood biochemistry (to detect e.g. electrolyte disturbances, hypo-albuminaemia) and liver function tests should also be carried out.

A chest radiograph (PA) supplemented by a lateral film is useful, in order to look for hilar masses (e.g. hilar nodes, bronchogenic carcinoma) causing dysphagia. A barium swallow (to outline the oesophagus) and meal (to examine the stomach) should be used to look for mucosal irregularity and abnormal contours. Ultrasound scanning may be useful for examining the liver and upper abdominal masses.

Upper gastrointestinal endoscopy (which many would contend should be carried out after a barium swallow has excluded a high obstructing oesophageal lesion) has the advantage that the mucosa can be directly visualized, and brushings or biopsies can be taken to investigate oesophagitis, Barrett's oesophagus, neoplasms or candidal infection. Upper endoscopy can also be used therapeutically, and dilatation of a stricture or the intubation of a neoplastic stricture may restore the ability to swallow fluids and food.

Abdominal pain*

Key points

- The 10 features of pain point to the likely diagnosis.

Patients with abdominal pain make great exam subjects from the examiners' point of view, because they can lead to discussion of so many different facets of surgery and medicine.

History

The history is all-important in determining the likely cause of the abdominal pain. After a thorough history has been taken, you will be able to produce a differential diagnosis for the cause of the pain in most patients.

The age and gender of the patient form a good starting point for the determination of the likely disease processes going on. Remember the 10 features of pain:

- site (ask the patient to point with one finger; has the site of pain changed?)
- severity (compared to previous experiences)
- characteristics (e.g. sharp, burning, gnawing, dull)
- radiation (e.g. to back, around abdominal wall, into groin)
- onset (e.g. sudden, gradual, time of day)
- periodicity (over minutes, hours)
- relieving factors (e.g. movement, vomiting, lying still, leaning forwards)
- exacerbating factors (e.g. movement, drinking fluids)
- associated features (e.g. nausea, vomiting, changes in the colour of urine, stool or skin)
- previous episodes (hours/days/weeks/years ago; more/less severe; diagnosis then?).

This information will help to direct you to which system is involved, but do not forget to complete the history and systematic enquiry – there may be important features, such as past medical illnesses, previous operations, previous and current medications or medical conditions (e.g. chronic pulmonary disease, cardiovascular disease), which may influence the patient's fitness for surgery.

Beware: pain perceived to be in the abdomen may be referred to the upper abdomen from organs superior to the diaphragm, particularly the heart (e.g. with angina or myocardial infarction) or the lung and pleurae (e.g. in pneumonia, lung infarction). In the case of women, do not forget the gynaecological causes of abdominal pain, including pelvic inflammatory disease, endometriosis and ovarian cyst rupture. Rare conditions (at least in surgical finals) which may present with abdominal pain include coeliac disease and irritable bowel syndrome (shortened to IBS, causing potential confusion with inflammatory bowel disease if you are not careful). IBS does, however, affect up to 25% of the general population.

Examination

Inspection, palpation, percussion and auscultation of the gastrointestinal system are required. These include examination of the hands, head and neck, mouth and abdomen. In addition you may need to examine the cardiorespiratory system if you think that the pain is referred from superior to the diaphragm.

If the physical examination and investigations are unremarkable, psychological assessment may be worthwhile but probably not in an exam setting!

Investigation

Investigations should begin with the urine and faeces, for signs of disease processes. A full blood count and biochemistry, plain abdominal radiograph, and ultrasound scan (particularly valuable for gallstones) complete the first-line investigations.

The symptoms and signs may point towards the upper gastro-intestinal tract, suggesting upper gastrointestinal endoscopy (with biopsy for *Helicobacter pylori*) or barium studies; or to the lower gastrointestinal tract, suggesting colonoscopy or barium studies.

Coeliac disease is diagnosed after duodenal biopsy and the detection of antigliadin antibodies. /endoyestal Crohn

Inflammatory bowel disease*

Key points

- Inflammatory bowel disease may affect multiple systems
- Remember the patient is an individual – how do their symptoms affect them?

History

Patients with inflammatory bowel disease often have a complex history, and many have had multiple hospital admissions and may have had several surgical operations. Fortunately, most patients are well versed in the chronology of their disease, the manage-ment of complications (such as obstruction, fistulae, stomata), and the medications they are on or have taken in the past. Complexity can make for a rambling history. When you present the patient to your examiners, make sure you have the key events clear: diagnosis and how it was made; attempts at medical treat-ment; and surgical procedures – what was done, when and why.

State how the disease has affected that individual – not only the symptoms of pain, diarrhoea etc. but also whether it has meant giving up work, missing time from college or university, significantly curtailing social activities.

Remember that patients with inflammatory bowel disease can also have one or more systemic manifestations, affecting the skin, eyes, joints and hepatobiliary system. Also, different parts of the intestinal tract may be affected at different times, particularly in Crohn's disease. There may be a family history of inflammatory bowel disease or bowel cancer (malignant change occurring in the context of inflammatory bowel disease).

Examination

On inspection, look for signs of malnutrition or anaemia (due to blood loss, or to vitamin B_{12} malabsorption as a result of terminal ileum malfunction or resection) and for signs of skin disease (e.g. erythema nodosum). Crohn's disease in particular can give rise to signs from the lips at one end to the perianal skin at the other, so you will need to examine both ends of the gastrointestinal tract, and all that lies between the two, where you can.

Abdominal examination may be complicated by the presence of a scar or a stoma (and sometimes more than one of each). The patient will often know exactly what type of stoma it is and allow you to confirm the presence of a spout (indicating an ileostomy). Multiple scars (which may be in unusual sites, and sometimes quite distorted due to postoperative sepsis) and fistulae (communications between two surfaces lined by epithelium) can also make abdominal examination difficult. It can be helpful, in a long case, to make a sketch of what you see and find, to refer to or to show to the examiners.

Investigation

A basic full blood count (to detect anaemia, which may be microcytic due to iron deficiency, or macrocytic) and blood biochemistry should be obtained, including liver function tests to detect biliary involvement. Trace element measurement (e.g. zinc, selenium) may be required if the patient is chronically malnourished. Markers of inflammation, including ESR and C-reactive protein, may be useful as indicators of disease activity.

Radiological investigations should include plain abdominal films (in the acute situation for loops of bowel, toxic dilation of the colon or bowel obstruction). Contrast studies can provide useful information. A small-bowel enema (the patient swallows a nasoenteric tube, down which contrast is injected) or small-bowel follow-through (after the patient has had a drink of contrast) can be used to examine the small intestine for strictures and fistulae. A colorectal double-contrast enema can provide useful information about colonic strictures, mucosal abnormalities or fistulae to other parts of the bowel or bladder.

Endoscopic examination may include upper gastrointestinal endoscopy, small bowel enteroscopy (if available) and colonoscopy. Colonoscopic screening of patients with long-standing ulcerative colitis should be considered because of the cancer risk. Patients with perianal Crohn's disease are particularly prone to fistulae and abscess formation, and so may require an examination under anaesthesia for adequate assessment of anorectal disease.

There is great overlap between ulcerative colitis and Crohn's disease, hence we have lumped them together but examiners will often ask about the differences between these two conditions. Table 8.1 will remind you of some of the key differences.

Table 8.1 Key differences between ulcerative colitis and Crohn's disease

	Ulcerative colitis	Crohn's disease
Age group	Generally 18–40 years	Bimodal 18–30+ >65 years
Site	Incontinuity proximally from the rectum	Skip lesions affecting any part of the GI tract Classically terminal ileum
Presentation	PR bleeding and diarrhoea	Dependent upon site
Radiology	Loss of haustral pattern and shallow ulcers on barium enema Plain films may show acute dilatation in emergency presentation	Rose thorn ulcers on barium enema Strictures and fistulae Distribution as above

Pancreatitis*

Key points

- Acute pancreatitis is usually secondary to gallstones or alcohol
- Diagnosis by elevated amylase ($> 3 \times$ normal)
- There are prognostic criteria for the severity of acute pancreatitis.
- Treatment is largely supportive

Pancreatitis can be classified as acute, recurrent/relapsing or chronic. Of acute cases 80% will resolve spontaneously without problems, but the 20% of patients who develop severe pancreatitis or complications are often seriously ill. A minority of patients will develop chronic pancreatitis, and others will have recurrent attacks of acute pancreatitis, being well between exacerbations. Recurrent attacks may occur because the agent responsible for the pancreatitis (e.g. alcohol) persists. Table 8.2 lists the causes of pancreatitis.

Table 8.2 Causes of pancreatitis	
Frequency of occurrence	Cause
Common (80% of cases in the UK)	Gallstones Alcohol
Intermediate	Trauma (post-ERCP; blunt abdominal trauma) Tumour (ampullary or pancreatic) Drugs (e.g. azathioprine, beta-blockers, steroids) Infection (e.g. viruses, particularly mumps) Hyperlipidaemia Hypothermia
Rare	Metabolic (e.g. hypercalcaemia) Congenital (e.g. pancreas divisum)
10% of cases	Idiopathic
(Mention scorpion sting to your examiners at your peril)	

If you have a patient with pancreatitis in surgical finals you should endeavour to:

- find the aetiological agent
- define the pattern of the patient's disease
- assess the severity of the attack.

The cause of the pancreatitis, and whether the patient is recovering from acute pancreatitis or has chronic pancreatitis, may be evident from the history. The most life-threatening complications of acute pancreatitis include renal failure, respiratory failure and cardiac failure, in addition to the necrosis (with or without supervening haemorrhage or sepsis) that may occur in the pancreatic bed. Malnutrition and opiate dependence are common complications of chronic pancreatitis.

History

Ask about pain, which is classically epigastric, radiating to the back and, in the acute situation, alleviated by leaning forwards or pacing around. In acute pancreatitis, the pain and rigid abdomen may mimic a perforated viscus. The pain may be exacerbated by precipitating factors (particularly alcohol), may be associated with nausea and vomiting and may only be relieved by strong (opioid) analgesia. Record the number of painful episodes, and find out whether the pain resolves completely between attacks.

In the case of chronic pancreatitis, particular questions should be asked about malabsorption (weight loss, stool difficult to flush away and offensive); diabetes (usually insulin-dependent); use of analgesics; previous investigations (such as ultrasound scanning, ERCP and CT scanning); and previous surgery.

It is important to try to determine the cause of the pancreatitis (usually gallstones or alcohol), and so questions must be asked about previous and current alcohol intake. A history of biliary colic, with or without jaundice and with or without fever, may suggest that gallstones are the underlying cause. The patient's occupation should be noted, particularly if it gives easy access to alcohol.

Examination

With the patient adequately exposed, look for signs of jaundice, bruising, or malnutrition (due to alcohol abuse, pancreatic insufficiency or chronic liver disease). Some of these signs may be evident on examination of the hands and torso, but examination of the abdomen will yield much more information. Inspection of the abdomen may reveal an abdominal mass (e.g. a pseudocyst or carcinoma). There may be scars from previous biliary or pancreatic surgery, but there will obviously be no evidence of ERCP. There may be drains, either to drain the pancreatic bed or to drain a pleural effusion secondary to the pancreatic inflammation. There may be a feeding tube passing into the jejunum, or a gastrostomy drainage tube to the stomach. Look for bruising (although neither the classical Cullen's periumbilical bruising nor Grey–Turner's flank bruising of acute pancreatitis are likely to be present in a patient used for exams). There may be signs of portal hypertension (e.g. caput medusae).

Ask whether the abdomen is tender or sore, and if so be particularly gentle when examining these areas. Palpate for hepatomegaly, splenomegaly, a pancreatic pseudocyst and pancreatic carcinoma, either of the latter two usually being palpable as a central abdominal mass. It is worth listening for a succussion splash, in case there is gastric outflow obstruction.

Percussion may confirm a mass, but auscultation with a stethoscope in surgical finals is unlikely to be useful in the abdominal examination. However, auscultation of the chest may demonstrate the side(s), size and extent of a unilateral or bilateral pleural effusion and the associated pulmonary features, particularly in a patient recovering from acute pancreatitis.

Investigation

The aims of the investigations are to establish the diagnosis of pancreatitis, assess its severity and suggest the appropriate therapy. The diagnosis and early prognostic criteria in acute pancreatitis may be based on: testing blood and urine for hyperamylasaemia ($3 \times$ the upper limit of normal; useful in diagnosis only); high blood glucose level; renal impairment; abnormal liver function tests; poor arterial blood oxygenation; a raised white cell count; anaemia; and abnormal coagulation (see Table 8.3). Beware that ischaemic bowel, acute cholecystitis or a perforated duodenal ulcer can also lead to hyperamylasaemia.

Useful information may be obtained from a chest radiograph (particularly in the case of pleural effusions) or from ultrasound scanning (for gallstones in particular, although the pancreas and

Table 8.3   **Early prognostic criteria for severity of acute pancreatitis**

Criterion	Threshold
Age of patient	>55 years
White blood cells	$>15 \times 10^9$/l
Glucose (in blood)	>10 mmol/l
Urea	>16 mmol/l
Pao_2	<8 kPa
Calcium	<2.0 mmol/l
Albumin	<32 g/l
LDH (lactate dehydrogenase)	>600 iu/l
ALT (alanine aminotransferase)	>100 u/l

any pseudocyst may be visualized). A plain abdominal film may demonstrate gas/fluid levels associated with ileus due to the pancreatitis. Also useful in appropriate circumstances is CT scanning (with contrast enhancement) to assess the swelling and necrosis of an acutely inflamed pancreas or to visualize one or more pseudocysts, an atrophic pancreas or a pancreatic carcinoma. Portal hypertension, in chronic alcoholic pancreatitis associated with alcoholic liver disease, may also be apparent from a CT scan. ERCP with sphincterotomy, to remove a stone obstructing the ampulla of Vater, or to assess the anatomy of the pancreatic duct in chronic pancreatitis, may also be useful.

Pancreatic exocrine insufficiency may be suggested by offensive, putty-like, yellow stool, and can be confirmed by measuring faecal fat content (with the patient on a suitable diet) or by the pancreatolauryl test (for pancreatic esterase activity). Pancreatic endocrine function can be assessed by a glucose tolerance test, if the patient is not overtly diabetic.

Management

The treatment of acute pancreatitis is conservative unless there are specific complications. Treatment should be as follows: analgesics (many prefer pethidine, which is said to cause least spasm of the sphincter of Oddi); fluid replacement (patients should be fasted and will require maintenance intravenous fluids, but in addition may have large nasogastric aspirates and peritoneal exudates); and monitoring, to ensure that complications are detected and treated promptly. Patients with severe disease warrant high-dependency type care. Patients may need physiotherapy because of pain and bed rest. Some will develop ARDS (acute respiratory distress syndrome) and will need ventilatory support.

Patients with severe pancreatitis who do not improve rapidly should be considered for ERCP and sphincterotomy if common bile duct stones are confirmed. A minority of patients will develop a pancreatic abscess or a pseudocyst, in which case percutaneous or surgical drainage of necrotic/infected material or a mature cyst may be needed.

The long-term care of patients with acute pancreatitis should be aimed at preventing further attacks. This may involve a cholecyst-ectomy if gallstones have been implicated as the causative agent, or it may involve emphatic advice about drinking habits or altering medications.

The management of chronic pancreatitis is a more long-term problem. Obviously every attempt should be made to remove aetiological factors. In addition, patients may need analgesics, insulin replacement and pancreatic extracts on a long-term basis. Surgery may be required for patients with intractable pain, and may involve either decompression of an obstructed pancreatic duct or resection of the pancreas. The latter will, however, condemn the patient to long-term insulin and pancreatic extract replacement therapy.

Rectal bleeding*

Key points

- The history will suggest the likely diagnosis
- Investigation of rectal bleeding aims to exclude life-threating conditions

For the purposes of surgical finals, rectal bleeding is most commonly due to haemorrhoids, carcinoma, polyps, diverticular disease, inflammatory bowel disease or angiodysplasia.

History

The key questions about rectal bleeding concern the colour of the blood and when the blood is seen. In general, bright red blood is rectal/anal in origin, dark blood is colonic and melaena signals blood from the proximal gastrointestinal tract. Fresh red blood on toilet paper only is likely to be from haemorrhoids; red blood on the stool is likely to be from a rectal lesion; and red or dark blood mixed in with the stool is likely to be from a colonic lesion. Bleeding due to diverticular disease may be sudden and profuse, but may stop spontaneously.

A previous history of dull left iliac fossa pain in a patient who has rectal bleeding may indicate diverticular disease. The colicky pain of bowel obstruction associated with blood in the stool may be due to a carcinoma. Pain on defaecation is a classic symptom of an anal fissure, which may result in a small amount of fresh blood on the stool and toilet paper. There may be mucus production (e.g. from a rectal adenoma) or blood/faecal staining of underwear (from haemorrhoids). Important symptoms which may be associated with bleeding are a change in bowel habit, or the recent onset of constipation or diarrhoea, any of which may occur with colorectal cancer or diverticular disease.

Ask about complications, e.g. colovesical fistula, which may present as recurrent urinary tract infections, dirty-coloured urine or (rarely) classic pneumaturia. Also ask about septic episodes and hospital admissions. A history of surgery for a polyp (usually performed via a colonoscope), for a cancer or previously for haemorrhoids or a fissure is worth noting.

A family history of colorectal cancer, polyps or inflammatory bowel disease is also important.

Examination

While taking a history, you may be able to assess whether a patient shows outward signs of systemic disease, such as cachexia.

Abdominal examination, of an appropriately positioned and exposed patient, should follow the scheme already outlined, with particular attention paid on inspection to scars, stomata and visible masses.

A diverticular mass or a tumour mass may be palpable. The colon, containing faeces, may be palpable proximal to a segment of diverticular disease or a colonic neoplasm. Remember to palpate for the liver, particularly if you suspect a colonic cancer.

Percussion should be used to confirm the resonance or dullness of any mass that you can palpate, and to help delineate the position of the liver.

Investigation

Dipstick testing of the urine may detect blood and protein. If there is a colovesical fistula, urine cultures grow gut organisms.

A full blood count may detect a microcytic anaemia if there is sufficient chronic blood loss. If there is ongoing inflammation, the white cell count may be raised.

However, the key investigations are endoscopic examination of the anal canal (proctoscopy), rectum (sigmoidoscopy) and colon (colonoscopy) or barium enema, followed by ultrasound scanning of the abdomen (supplemented by CT scanning) to detect liver metastases or inflammatory masses.

Abdominal aortic aneurysm†

Key points

- Back/loin pain mimicking renal colic ± a hypotensive episode in an elderly patient is suggestive of a leaking abdominal aortic aneurysm.

Most aneurysms are degenerative in origin and associated with atherosclerotic disease elsewhere in the cardiovascular system. Inflammatory aneurysms are comparatively rare (if you touch on this topic in your exam, immunological tests for syphilis may be mentioned).

History

An abdominal aortic aneurysm may be asymptomatic, or may cause back pain. A leaking aneurysm may present with back pain or loin pain, a history of collapse or a hypotensive episode in the acute context (beware when examining an elderly patient who has collapsed with 'renal colic' – he or she may well have a leaking abdominal aortic aneurysm). If you have the opportunity (e.g. in a long case), ask whether the patient has any other history of peripheral, cardiac or cerebral vascular disease, and whether he or she is a smoker.

Examination

Remember to seek features of peripheral vascular disease on inspection (e.g. skin changes, ulceration, ischaemia, gangrene, amputation), palpation (pulses) and auscultation (bruits).

On abdominal examination, an aortic aneurysm is a mass which is expansile, centrally positioned (though it may be more prominent on the left-hand or right-hand side) and, sometimes, tender. Normal aortic pulsation may be visible on inspection, and may be readily palpable in a thin, normal, person. In an elderly person the aorta may be ectatic, and it may be difficult to be sure it is not aneurysmal.

Palpate the aorta using two digits, as described earlier, to delineate the extent of the expansile abdominal mass.

Auscultate for a bruit over the aorta, iliac vessels and renal arteries.

Investigation

A plain radiograph/lateral film of the abdomen may show the calcified wall of the aneurysm. However, an ultrasound scan should allow accurate measurement of the size and extent of the aneurysm, including any extension into the iliac vessels or proximal to the renal vessels. Increasing size, particularly over 5 cm, leads to a greater chance of leakage from or rupture of the aneurysm.

Splenomegaly[†]

Splenomegaly may be caused by: portal hypertension/occlusion; haematological causes, e.g. lymphoma (causing fever, weight loss and lymph node enlargement), leukaemia (particularly CLL (chronic lymphocytic leukaemia)), myelofibrosis; Felty's syndrome (with rheumatoid arthritis); or infective causes (particularly Epstein–Barr virus and malaria). Occasionally, patients with a large spleen turn up in the exam – the most likely causes of splenomegaly in this situation are CLL, myelofibrosis or infection.

History

Remember to ask about family history, travel abroad and infective contacts.

Examination

Distinguishing between the spleen and the left kidney may depend on the presence of a splenic notch, a dull percussion note overlying the mass, and the position of the spleen close to the costal margin (you cannot 'get above' the spleen, i.e. insert your fingers between the spleen and the costal margin). Both the spleen and the kidney move on inspiration, but the spleen may appear to move infero-medially and the kidney inferiorly only.

In most surgical splenomegaly cases, the spleen is just palpable.

Investigation

The key investigations are haematological (including blood films) and ultrasound scanning.

SUMMARY

There are some diagnoses and problems which come up with regularity in surgical finals. Table 8.4 lists the most common conditions, their typical features (not all of which have to be present in every patient) and one key investigation (although other investigations may also be helpful).

Table 8.4 Common abdominal cases

Condition	Typical features	Key diagnostic investigation
Biliary colic	Upper abdominal pain, increasing to plateau and dispersing after a few hours; may be described as a band around the upper (right) abdomen	Ultrasound
Pancreatitis	*Acute:* severe epigastric pain, radiating to back; may imitate perforated ulcer	Serum/urine amylase
	Chronic: persistent abdominal/back pain, with exacerbations; features of pancreatic insufficiency	ERCP
Peptic ulcer	Dyspepsia; epigastric pain, worse or relieved on eating; patient wakens at night	Upper endoscopy
Renal colic	Severe right/left-sided pain, radiating to the groin/testicle	Intravenous urogram
Colonic neoplasm	Rectal bleeding; anaemia; mucus; change in bowel habit	Colonscopy
Diverticular disease	Left iliac fossa pain; pellet stools; diarrhoea/constipation; rectal bleeding	Barium enema
Bowel obstruction	Abdominal distension; colicky pain; vomiting	Plain radiograph

Key questions

1. What are causes of, and how would you investigate:
   - jaundice?
   - altered bowel habit?
   - rectal bleeding?
   - hepatomegaly?
   - ascites?
   - a mass in the right upper quadrant?
   - a mass in the left upper quadrant?
   - a mass in the right iliac fossa?
   - a mass in the left iliac fossa?
   - a central abdominal mass?
2. What problems might be encountered when operating on a jaundiced patient?
3. How would you assess a patient with dysphagia?
4. What are the differences between Crohn's disease and ulcerative colitis?
5. What are the features and complications of acute pancreatitis?

9

Hernias and the groin

A hernia is an abnormal protrusion of an organ or tissue from its normal body cavity or restraining sheath. In surgical finals, hernias of the abdominal wall are very common short cases (particularly in the groin, in the midline or associated with incisions), since they are suitable for examination by several candidates. A patient in a long case may have a hiatus hernia along with other conditions.

Abdominal hernias have a peritoneal sac, which passes through a defect in the abdominal wall. A small, tight, hernial orifice (the neck of the sac) may result in a hernia which is irreducible (rather than reducible) and the contents may become obstructed (e.g. the bowel) or strangulated (e.g. fat, omentum or bowel). Strangulation (compromise of the blood supply to the contents of the hernial sac) results from venous occlusion, then arterial occlusion and consequent gangrene. Not surprisingly, morbidity and mortality follow.

Other categories of hernia include paraumbilical, epigastric and incisional.

There are two favourite kinds of hernia which come up in exams. One is the sliding hernia, in which an organ forms part of the hernia wall and may be damaged during surgery (such as the bladder in the medial wall of a direct inguinal hernia). The other is Richter's hernia, in which strangulation of part of the circumference of the bowel wall occurs, but with sufficient bowel outwith the hernia, so that there is no bowel obstruction.

Key points

- A small, tight, hernial orifice is more likely to entrap protuding organs than is a wide neck to the hernia sac

TYPICAL CASES

Groin hernias*

Key points

- Determine whether this is a femoral, direct inguinal or indirect inguinal hernia
- Is it reducible?
- Is it a recurrent hernia?

The anatomy of the inguinal region is a favourite subject with examiners, and is well worth revising (see Figs 9.1 and 9.2). Examiners also like to test you on the differences between indirect inguinal, direct inguinal and femoral hernias: these may matter in clinical practice, because indirect inguinal hernias and (particularly) femoral hernias are prone to strangulation. However, it can sometimes be difficult to tell one from another, so a few hints are given in Table 9.1.

History

The history of a groin swelling or a hernia should include the patient's age and occupation and a history of the swelling. Ask when the swelling first appeared, and whether it has changed in

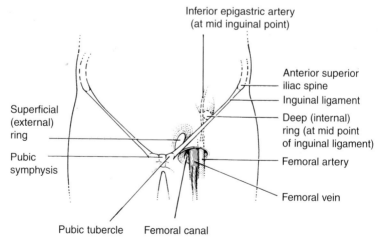

Fig. 9.1 Anatomy of the inguinal region

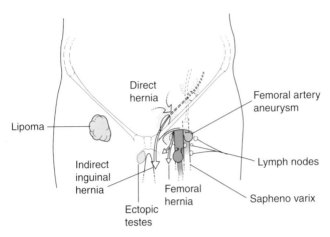

Fig. 9.2 Groin swellings

Table 9.1	Features of inguinal and femoral hernias		
Features	Indirect inguinal hernia	Direct inguinal hernia	Femoral hernia
Typical patient	Younger male	Older male	Old female
Proportion of groin hernias	60%	25%	15%
Anatomy	Commences at deep ring, lateral to the inferior epigastric artery, and passes within the coverings of the spermatic cord	Bulges medial to the inferior epigastric artery	Emerges from the femoral canal
Relationship to the public tubercle	Starts lateral to and above the tubercle, but passes superomedial to the tubercule into the scrotum	Lies above the tubercle	Passes inferolateral to the tubercle
Descends into the scrotum?	Yes	No	No
Obstructs or strangulates?	Yes	Rarely	Yes

size or is tender. In the case of a hernia, can it be pushed back (always, sometimes or only when lying down)? Does the patient have any history of conditions which could result in increased intra-abdominal pressure, such as a chronic cough, constipation, symptoms of prostatic outflow obstruction or ascites? Is there only one hernia, or has the patient noticed another?

Some patients have had previous hernia surgery, on the same side (so the hernia may be recurrent) or on the opposite side. They will know whether the hernia repair was performed as a child (when simple excision of the sac, herniotomy, will have been performed), or as an emergency or elective procedure. Until recently, hernia repair was performed by open surgery using sutures, but laparoscopic hernia repair and the use of prosthetic mesh have now become popular.

Examination

Key points

- Full exposure of the groin
- Examine the patient stably and lying down

Examination should follow the standard routine of exposure/inspection, palpation, percussion and auscultation.

It is traditional to examine the patient lying down first and then standing, as some small indirect or direct hernias are only detectable when a patient is standing. Remember to ask your examiner if you can examine the patient when standing. Full exposure of the groin area (including the scrotum in men) is needed to examine for hernias. Look first for surgical scars of open or laparoscopic hernia surgery: this can be more difficult than might be thought, because an old skin crease incision can heal almost to invisibility, and may be camouflaged by pubic hair. Visually identify any hernial orifices, and ask the patient to cough. Remember to look at both sides.

With the patient lying down, identify the palpable anatomical landmarks:

- the pubic tubercle
- the anterior superior iliac spine
- the femoral pulsation.

Now gently palpate the hernia and determine:

- its position relative to the pubic tubercle (inguinal superior, femoral inferior)

- if it is reducible (many candidates try to reduce the hernia with the patient standing – this is fruitless and will cause pain to the patient)
- if it is an inguinal hernia, whether it is direct or indirect:
  direct
      sac superior and lateral to pubic tubercle
      not controlled by pressure over the internal ring
  indirect
      sac passes obliquely into scrotum, therefore superior and medial to pubic tubercle
      controlled by pressure over the internal ring (above the mid point of the inguinal ligament; superolateral to the femoral pulse).
- if there is a contralateral hernia.

Percussion over a large hernia containing a hollow viscus (e.g. small bowel, colon) will be tympanic, while percussion of the omentum will not.

On auscultation over a hernia you may hear bowel sounds. You can comment on whether they sound normal (most likely in an exam) or obstructive (runs of high-pitched sounds), or are absent.

Other hernias

The locations of various types of hernia are shown in Figure 9.3. All hernias should be gently manipulated to assess reducibility. Ask the patient whether the hernia can be reduced, and enlist his or her help if you are allowed. Identify the margins of the hernial orifice: strangulation is less likely in the case of a large defect than if the sac has a small tight neck. If the hernia is reducible, try to control the neck of the sac and ask the patient to cough again.

Incisional hernias*

Key points

- Incisional hernias are often associated with previous wound complications
- Large diffuse hernias may be awkward to deal with but remember to determine whether it is reducible or not and to define the margins.

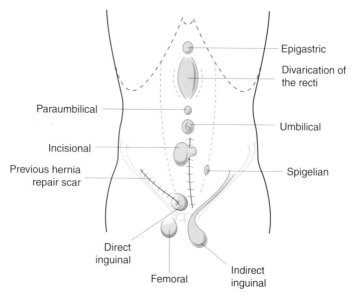

Fig. 9.3 Location of hernias

History

Ask the patient about any previous operation(s), and about any associated complications such as wound infection or dehiscence, which may have predisposed to the development of an incisional hernia. Are there any underlying medical conditions which may predispose to raised intra-abdominal pressure or impaired wound healing? A heavy lifting job may have contributed to the development of an incisional hernia.

Examination

With the patient fully exposed, following inspection comment on the position of the surgical scar(s) and the swelling due to the hernia. The hernia often appears lateral to a mid-line wound – this may indicate a button-holing through a suture or simply be due to the way it has expanded. Is the hernia reducible? If so, when the patient lies down and relaxes the hernia will reduce, whereas if asked to cough or tense up the abdominal muscles (by lifting his head off the pillow or raising a straightened leg), the hernia will become obvious. Alternatively the hernia may be incarcerated and impossible to reduce fully. Attempt to define the neck of the hernia, and determine whether it is wide or narrow.

Treatment

Treatment of an incisional hernia is surgical, by reopening and resuturing the wound or by suturing a mesh over the defect. Remember that the repair of a large incisional hernia can significantly increase intra-abdominal pressure, and lead to respiratory embarrassment.

Umbilical and paraumbilical hernias

True umbilical hernias occur in infants and are a hernia through a weakened umbilical scar. Usually the hernia will improve spontaneously and there is little risk of strangulation.

In adults hernias around the unbilicus occur not through the umbilical scar but as a protrusion through the lineas alba just above or just below the umbilicus (para-umbilical hernia). These may be relatively small protrusions or large sacs.

Other groin swellings

Lumps in the groin which are inferior to the inguinal ligament but not in the scrotum (see Fig. 9.2) can pose a problem in surgical finals. These lumps include inguinal nodes (usually multiple, and may be bilateral), sapheno varix (compressible, with a cough impulse), lipoma, femoral artery aneurysm, ectopic testis and psoas abscess (the latter uncommon). The sites of various types of scrotal swelling are depicted in Figure 9.4.

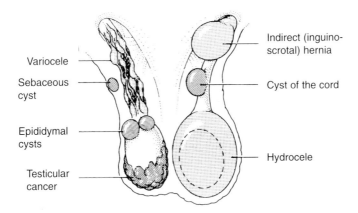

Fig. 9.4 Scrotal swellings

History

Do not forget that the external genitalia, perineum and anal area form part of a surgical patient's abdominal examination. Specific points in the history should include any previous surgery (e.g. for a hernia, or to the testes or scrotum, including vasectomy) and any history of sexually-transmitted conditions, together with the duration of any testicular swelling and any changes in size or shape of the testes.

Examination

Key points

- Ultrasound examination is very useful to aid diagnosis of scrotal swellings

In men, scars in the groin or on the scrotum can be extremely difficult to identify. Check that there are two testes and ask of any scrotal swelling:

- can you feel that the testis is separate from the lump (e.g. epididymal cyst, cyst of the cord or hernia)?
- can you palpate above the lump? (If so, it may be a true testicular swelling, an epididymal cyst or a hydrocele; if not, it may be an indirect inguinal hernia.)
- can you transilluminate the lump? (If so, it is fluid-filled and likely to be a hydrocele.)

Investigation

The key investigation for groin and testicular swellings is ultrasound scanning, which can clearly delineate the various pathologies. You may be asked about tumour markers (e.g. beta-HCG (human chorionic gonadotrophin), AFP (alpha fetoprotein)) if a testicular cancer is suspected.

Hydrocele*

Key points

- A hydrocele may be primary (idiopathic or congenital) or secondary to disease of the testis (testicular cancer, epididymal orchitis)

A hydrocele is common in surgical finals. It may be several cm in size, but is confined to the scrotum (one can 'get above it'). The testis cannot be palpated separately from the swelling, and it should be possible to transilluminate the swelling. Hydroceles may be bilateral.

Epididymal cyst*

Key points

- An epididymal cyst is palpable separate from the testis

An epididymal cyst is usually about 1 cm in size, and found at the upper pole of the testis. Epididymal cysts may be single or multiple, unilateral or bilateral, and may be tender.

Varicocele[†]

Key points

- With the patient standing a varicocele resembles a bag of worms

A varicocele is most commonly identified simply by inspecting the scrotum with the patient standing, when the prominent veins (claimed to resemble a bag of worms) will be apparent. A varicocele is said to be more common on the left-hand side (due to the drainage of the left testicular vein into the left renal vein). In an older man, a varicocele of recent onset may be the first outward sign of a renal cancer (again due to the venous drainage).

Testicular tumours[§]

True testicular lumps are uncommon in finals, and are likely to be testicular tumours. Testicular tumours may, nevertheless, be discussed as part of the differential diagnosis.

Ectopic testis[§]

An ectopic testis is unusual in surgical finals. It is often associated with an inguinal hernia. Beware the absent testis (due to maldescent, ectopia or surgical removal).

Other conditions

The skin of the groin can harbour any of the lumps and bumps described in Chapter 4. Sebaceous cysts are particularly common. Squamous carcinoma of the scrotum, beloved of older textbooks, is no longer a likely short case as the days of the child chimney-sweep are long gone. However, squamous carcinoma of the penis is a possible short case and you *must* examine beneath the foreskin of an uncircumcized man (ask the patient to retract his foreskin, or wear gloves to retract it yourself).

In the perianal area, inspect for papillomata (warts, which are common), an abscess or consequent fistula (if there is recurrent perianal sepsis, think of Crohn's disease), or anal carcinoma (a ragged ulcer with a bloody necrotic discharge).

Regional lymph nodes from the glans, the penile and scrotal skin and the anus are in the groin. Therefore infection or tumour growth will be reflected in these nodes. The lymphatic drainage from the testes is intra-abdominal to para-aortic nodes.

Key questions

1. What are the differences between indirect inguinal, direct inguinal and femoral hernias?
2. What is the difference between an incarcerated and a strangulated hernia?
3. Is a narrow or a wide neck to a hernial sac more dangerous?
4. What is a sliding hernia?
5. How would you distinguish an indirect inguinal hernia in the scrotum from a hydrocele?
6. How would you distinguish an epididymal cyst from a hydrocele?
7. What lesions other than hernias, hydroceles and epididymal cysts can occur in the groin or perineum?
8. Where do the testicular lymph nodes drain to?

10

Limbs (vascular)

In surgical finals it is common for you to be asked to examine a patient's hand or comment on the lower limb. This may require you to think of several different systems, such as cardiovascular, locomotor and neurological, during the examination. There are many conditions that you may encounter, but your examination should follow the same general scheme as elsewhere: exposure/position, inspection, palpation, percussion and auscultation. For orthopaedic problems, this may be modified to: exposure/position, look, feel and move. This is simply a different way of performing inspection and palpation. Percussion has a reduced role in the examination of the limbs and back, but auscultation is important in vascular examination. Specific aspects of your examination of a patient will be more important for vascular problems than for orthopaedic problems and vice versa. This chapter highlights vascular cases, and the next chapter looks at orthopaedic problems likely to come up in surgical finals, although this division is somewhat artificial.

HISTORY

You may be asked 'Examine this woman's hands' or 'What do you think of this man's lower limbs?', which doesn't leave much scope for taking a history. However, you will be able to judge the approximate age of the patient and the gender. It is sometimes hard to miss the heavily nicotine-stained fingers or mouth of a heavy smoker, and you can impress your examiner by mentioning this (if given the chance). If you are permitted to ask questions, after establishing the age and (former) occupation of the patient, ask an open question such as 'What are the problems that brought you into hospital?' or 'What troubles do you get from your hands/legs?'.

Specific questions applicable to particular limb problems are outlined in each section below.

EXAMINATION

Exposure/position

Make sure that you can see the whole of the limb that you are supposed to be examining, and the contralateral limb as well. This means you will probably have to help the patient undress to expose the body parts you are interested in. Ensure that the patient is then lying (or sitting) comfortably so that you can proceed.

Inspection

Look at the patient's skin for discoloration, signs of trauma (including surgical scars), ulceration and gangrene. Look for deformities, swelling (joint or soft tissue) and muscle wasting. Ask the patient to lift up each limb to ensure that you are not missing something (such as a pressure sore on the heel). You may need to assist the patient, and do ask if the limb is sore before you touch or move it. You will usually be able to compare the limb you have been asked to examine with the contralateral limb, although amputees are a popular choice of patient for some surgical finals.

Palpation

Ask if the limb or joints are painful before you touch the patient, and watch his or her face during the examination to ensure that you are not causing distress. Feel the temperature of the two limbs (using the dorsum of your fingers, which is said to be the most sensitive part), examine the nails and assess capillary filling (blanch the nail with pressure from your finger, then see how long it takes for the colour to return). Palpate the major limb pulses, on the right and left sides.

Auscultation

Auscultation is normally confined to listening for bruits over the arterial tree, but take care that any bruit you hear is not transmitted from more proximal vessels which are diseased. Rarely, arterio-

venous malformations may appear in finals. Unless the arteriovenous connection is a surgically-manufactured fistula (usually in
the forearm, for access for dialysis), and so has a high flow rate, you
are unlikely to hear a bruit.

TYPICAL CASES

- arterial disease
  - occlusive[*]
  - aneurysmal[†]
  - arteriovenous fistula[§]
- venous disease
  - varicose veins[*]
  - venous thrombosis[†]
- lymphatic disease
  - primary lymphoedema[§]
  - secondary lymphoedema.[†]

Arterial disease*

Key points

- Claudication distance suggests the severity of arterial
  disease (shorter = more severe)
- The muscle groups affected indicates the likely site(s) of
  stenosis

Chronic arterial insufficiency secondary to atherosclerosis is almost
a certainty in surgical finals. The symptoms are usually worse in the
lower limbs than in the upper limbs, so patients used in exams
usually have lower limb problems. The following scheme for history
and examination is presented in terms of the lower limbs, but can
easily be modified for use in the context of the upper limbs.

History

Ask about specific symptoms due to arterial insufficiency, and
also carry out systematic enquiries about any cardiovascular
and respiratory symptoms.

The pain of claudication (pain develops on exercise and is relieved when exercise stops) indicates that the blood supply to the muscle(s) affected is inadequate to cope with exercise. It should be distinguished from sciatic nerve pain, which originates in the buttock, passes down the back of the leg to below the knee, and is associated with pain on raising a straight leg and with possible neurological signs. Ask about claudication distance (the distance at which the pain comes on). This is usually remarkably constant for walking either on the flat or up stairs. Ask whether the claudication distance is increasing, static or decreasing, and how the claudication affects daily living. Determine which muscle groups are affected by claudication, to indicate where the stenosis is situated:

- calf pain indicates stenosis of the superficial femoral/popliteal arteries
- thigh and calf pain indicate stenosis of the external iliac artery
- buttock, thigh and calf pain indicate stenosis of the external and internal iliac arteries
- bilateral lower limb pain indicates stenosis of the aorta.

Determine what treatment(s) the patient and his or her clinicians have tried. Rest pain in a limb is a sign of severe ischaemia, and of impending gangrene, as the arterial perfusion is inadequate even for the skin. Rest pain often occurs first in bed at night, when the limb is warm and perfusion pressure is lowered by the horizontal position – patients may gain relief by dangling the limb over the edge of the bed. This phenomenon can be used in clinical examination (Buerger's test) to assess the time of venous filling/reactive hyperaemia when the leg is dangled over the side of the bed.

Cardiac and respiratory disease may not only exacerbate arterial insufficiency but influence its possible management. Does the patient smoke (currently/previously/never; how many per day)? Is the patient diabetic, and if so, how is the diabetes controlled? Is there any history of ischaemic heart disease, cerebrovascular accident, chronic obstructive pulmonary disease, hypertension, hypercholesterolaemia, impotence, or a family history of vascular disease?

Examination

The limbs to be examined should be fully exposed: for examination of the lower limbs, the patient should wear only underwear from the waist down and for examination of the upper limbs, no shirt. Remember to expose both limbs so that they can be compared with each other. Patients may be most comfortable lying on a couch (where the lower limbs can readily be seen).

Although they may not obviously be part of an examination of the lower limb, the patient's pulse (rate, rhythm, regularity) and blood pressure (diastolic/systolic) should be recorded as part of a full cardiovascular assessement.

Look for obvious signs of loss of viability, such as shiny, atrophic skin; hair loss or atrophic nails (the latter two are not very specific signs, but should get a mention in exams); ulceration; or overt gangrene. Look to see if the limb is pale or has a red, hyperaemic glow and blanches on elevation. Remember to look at the pressure areas (the heel, the lateral border of the foot, the first metatarsal head and the malleoli), particularly in diabetics, and look between the toes.

Feel the temperature of the limb (use the dorsum of the fingers) at various levels, and compare it with that of the contralateral limb. Use gentle pressure to check for pitting oedema at the ankle (and more proximally, if it looks oedematous). Assess capillary return in the toe pulp: apply pressure for 2 seconds to blanch the capillary bed, then measure the capillary refill time. Palpate the peripheral pulses: femoral, popliteal (with the patient's knee flexed at 45°, use the pulps of your fingers of both hands to feel for the pulse), dorsalis pedis and posterior tibial. The scoring convention is: 0 (absent); +/− (reduced); 1 (normal); 2 (aneurysmal). Compare the pulses on the left with those on the right. Note the rate, rhythm and regularity, and check for radial/femoral delay.

Listen for bruits over the femoral arteries. Remember that occluded vessels will have no flow, and hence no bruit.

At the end of the history and examination, you should be able to:

- describe the patient's symptoms and signs
- comment on the way in which these affect his or her lifestyle
- say where the vascular tree is occluded.

Investigation

Test the urine for glucose (diabetes and peripheral vascular disease make a great combined medical and surgical long case).

Blood should be tested for anaemia or polycythaemia (both of which may worsen the symptoms of peripheral ischaemia); ESR (to suggest inflammatory causes of peripheral vascular disease); and biochemistry (to detect renal failure and extent of diabetic control).

An ECG and chest radiograph are useful in the assessment of the general health of patients with peripheral vascular disease, particularly if they are likely to benefit from interventional radiology or reconstructive surgery.

Noninvasive investigations include Doppler scanning, to detect blood flow and to measure the pulse pressures, enabling a comparison between the upper limb and lower limb pressures. If Doppler scanning is used to measure the ankle and brachial pressures, the ABPI (ankle/brachial pressure index) can be derived, with the following implications:

ABPI > 1.0 – normal
ABPI = 0.7–1.0 – claudication
ABPI = 0.4–0.7 – moderate ischaemia
ABPI < 0.4 – severe ischaemia.

Angiography may be considered to be the definitive investigation for arterial disease, as it provides a 'road map' of the patient's vessels, showing the level, length and severity of stenoses and occluded vessels. Angiography is performed by direct arterial puncture (under local anaesthetic) of the femoral artery, and since it is not without potential morbidity (e.g. haematoma, worsening the lower limb ischaemia, embolism of atheromatous plaque to the lower limb) it should be reserved for patients in whom surgical or radiological intervention is contemplated.

Angioscopy, in which the vascular anatomy and abnormalities are directly visualized, is an even more specialized investigation.

Management

The management and treatment options, as ever, are conservative measures, medical treatment or surgical treatment and the choice will vary according to the severity of the disease:

- mild/moderate claudication
  - stop smoking
  - lose weight
  - control diabetes
  - foot care
  - exercise
  - venesection if polycythaemic

- optimize medical treatment (of diabetes, cardiac function, etc.)
- disabling claudication
  - conservative and medical treatment (as above)
  - balloon angioplasty
  - reconstructive surgery
- critical limb ischaemia
  - conservative and medical therapy to optimize the patient's general condition
  - balloon angioplasty
  - reconstructive surgery
  - lumbar sympathectomy
  - amputation.

Gangrene*

Key points

- Dry (ischaemic) gangrene is secondary to peripheral vascular disease. Wet (infective) gangrene is secondary to bacterial infection

Dry gangrene (ischaemic), unlike wet gangrene (infective), is a common problem in finals.

The history should be as outlined for peripheral vascular disease. The patient may already have attempted reconstructive vascular surgery or interventional radiology.

On examination, the gangrenous areas may be very small (e.g. the tips of one or more toes), so remember to inspect the heel and between the toes thoroughly. Alternatively, the gangrene may be quite obvious (remember to look at the contralateral limb, which may already have required amputation). Obvious black, hard, gangrenous flesh may be surrounded by skin which is hyperaemic, red and shiny, but still ischaemic.

Atrial fibrillation*

The most common abnormal pulse you will be asked to feel in finals is that associated with atrial fibrillation, although you cannot say so straight away and spoil the examiners' fun! Technically, you should also require an ECG, which will demonstrate the absence of

P waves and an irregularly irregular pulse. Common causes of atrial fibrillation include ischaemic heart disease, posterior myocardial infarction, hyperthyroidism and rheumatic heart disease.

Acute limb ischaemia[†]

Although you are unlikely to meet a patient with acute limb ischaemia, which is a surgical emergency if the limb is to be saved, you may see a patient who has had surgery for acute limb ischaemia or get into a discussion on the topic after seeing a patient with chronic limb ischaemia. The symptoms and signs of acute ischaemia are known as the 'six Ps':

- pain
- pulseless
- pallor
- perishingly cold (a bit contrived!)
- paraesthesia
- powerless.

The first four of these features occur at the time of the acute ischaemic event (either embolic (which may be secondary to atrial fibrillation) or thrombosis on an atherosclerotic plaque), and the neurological effects afterwards.

The aim of treatment is to restore the circulation as soon as possible. If embolic occlusion is suspected, retrieval of the thrombus using a balloon (Fogarty) catheter can be attempted during surgical exploration of the artery, which should be followed by anti-coagulation using heparin. If this is unsuccessful, intraoperative angiography is needed. Alternatively, in patients where thrombosis in pre-existing arterial disease is suspected, the key investigation is angiography prior to surgery, with the option of lysis of the occluding thrombus. Potential complications include recurrence of the ischaemia (and new emboli?), loss of (part of) the limb, compartment syndrome and myoglobin-induced renal failure.

Amputations[†]

In contrast to upper limb amputations (which are usually traumatic in origin, and often involve one or more digits), amputations of the lower limb are usually surgical and secondary to vascular disease.

Amputations you may be shown in finals are described below, uncommon amputations are marked with an asterisk:

- hindquarter
  - amputation through the hip*
- above knee
  - amputation through the distal femur
  - prosthesis may be fitted
  - less mobility than for below knee
- through knee
  - amputation through the knee joint*
- below knee
  - tibia transected 10cm below the knee joint
  - knee joint retained
  - flexibility and mobility good
- Syme amputation
  - heel forms the stump: common in 19th century as a result of trauma*
- mid foot
  - through the tarsal/metatarsal junction*
- metatarsal
  - individual, usually fifth, metatarsal + digit
- digital
  - one or more digits.

Accompanying the amputation(s), there may be contractures or infected/incompletely healed amputation wounds. The patient may have a walking stick or prosthesis, or even be sitting in a wheelchair.

Diabetic foot[†]

The diabetic patient with lower limb disease may have many of the features already described above. The combination of neuropathy with arterial disease, and perhaps with infection, puts the lower limb (and particularly the foot) at risk. Patients with these conditions are usually comparatively young, with the pulses present and a warm (often infected) foot, and can be contrasted with an older patient with peripheral vascular disease, who has a cold, pulseless foot with dry gangrene.

Peripheral aneurysms[§]

Trauma (including iatrogenic trauma due to arterial puncture), atherosclerosis or inflammatory disease can weaken the wall of an artery, resulting in an aneurysm. Although the abdominal aortic aneurysm springs to mind first, you may also encounter in surgical finals a subclavian artery aneurysm (which may be associated with thoracic outlet compression); a femoral artery aneurysm (usually at the site of arterial puncture) or a popliteal artery aneurysm.

History

If you can take a full history as outlined above, all well and good. If you can only ask three questions (for example in a short case), ask if there is any history of smoking, diabetes (and preferably how it is controlled) or trauma.

Examination

Full exposure of the limb is once again important: this may reveal evidence of embolism to, and consequent ischaemia (or gangrene) of, the digits due to a subclavian aneurysm, or thrombosis due to a popliteal aneurysm (with distal ischaemia).

Inspection may reveal obvious pulsation in the line of the subclavian, femoral or popliteal artery. Unfortunately an ectatic artery in a thin, older person can appear at first sight to be an aneurysm (the carotid version of this is unkindly called a 'student's aneurysm' for that very reason). Hence palpation (to demonstrate an expansile lesion, the size of which can be measured) is required to establish the diagnosis.

An audible bruit may be apparent over or distal to the aneurysm, due to the disordered flow caused by the aneurysm.

Investigation

Angiography is the key investigation for peripheral aneurysms, but preparation of the patient for theatre will require in addition urinalysis, a full blood count, blood biochemistry, ECG, chest radiograph, etc. For an aortic aneurysm an ultrasound ± CT scan will be required to determine the relationship of the aneurysm to the renal vessels.

Treatment

Conventional surgical treatment usually involves bypassing the affected segment of the vessel, using a vein or synthetic graft, and tying off the aneurysm.

Arteriovenous malformations[§]

It is possible for an arteriovenous malformation to require an increased cardiac output and hence to cause a hyperdynamic circulation (with an aortic flow murmur), or even heart failure. Alternatively, the result may be limb hypertrophy or ulceration.

History

The duration of the lesion (has it been present since birth?), any history of trauma (surgical or otherwise) and any change in the size of the lesion or symptoms (e.g. discomfort) related to the malformation are important.

Examination

Adequately expose the lesion and the remainder of the limb (or torso, if the lesion is there). Inspection should allow you to comment on the position, size (in cm), shape, colour and contour of the lesion, and on any associated features such as scars (surgical or traumatic).

Next palpate the lesion for consistency, pulsation, compressibility, draining/filling on raising/lowering the limb, and thrill.

Then auscultate for a bruit (a continuous murmur).

Haemangioma[§]

A haemangioma can range in size from a few mm to a large, disfiguring lesion with associated increased growth of the ipsilateral limb, due to increased blood flow. A small haemangioma may contain thrombosed blood, and so have a bluish tinge and feel firm. If the outflow is intact, the haemangioma may feel soft and may empty with pressure. Haemangiomata are not usually fixed to deeper tissues, and rarely have a bruit (but you still need to listen, to please your examiner!).

Arteriovenous fistula[§]

In exams and hospital practice the common arteriovenous fistula is that which has been formed for dialysis access, usually at the wrist, antecubital fossa or ankle.

There may be visible venous filling (greater on the side with the fistula than on the contralateral side) and there will be a surgical scar, a palpable thrill and, on auscultation, an audible bruit.

Venous disease*

Key points

- Varicose veins follow sapheno-femoral and venous valve in–competence
- Varicose veins may follow deep venous thrombosis
- Varicose ulceration, consequent upon varicose veins, occurs proximal to the medial malleolus

Venous disease and (especially) varicose veins are common in finals, and make particularly good short cases. It will be assumed by every teacher and examiner you meet that you have seen hundreds of patients with varicose veins, so take the trouble to see such patients and examine them under supervision on the wards and in the Outpatient Department.

History

Questions, in addition to those about the patient's general health and fitness for surgery, should include the onset, distribution and symptoms from the veins. Their onset may be due to a problem with the deep venous system, so ask about deep venous thrombosis, pulmonary embolism and trauma to the lower limb. More commonly, varicose veins result from congenital saphenofemoral incompetence or occur during pregnancy. The distribution may sound as if it is related to the long saphenous vein or the short saphenous vein or perhaps both. Varicose veins often get blamed for all sorts of symptoms to which they are unrelated but skin itch, ache, bruising and ulceration may be mentioned.

Ask about previous surgery, involving a high tie (saphenofemoral ligation), venous stripping (of the great saphenous vein), multiple ligations or avulsions. Was surgery performed on the short saphenous system? Has there been a second or third operation? Has skin grafting been required for varicose ulceration?

Examination

Follow the standard exposure/position, inspection, palpation, percussion, (auscultation) scheme.

Having exposed both legs to the groin, varicose veins will be most readily demonstrated with the patient standing (see Fig. 10.1). Look at each lower limb in turn, and comment on the distribution of visible varicose veins to the long saphenous system (from the groin, the vein passes posteromedial to the knee joint, then anterior to the medial malleolus); the distribution of visible varicose veins to the short saphenous system (from the popliteal fossa, the vein passes inferiorly to the lateral border of the foot); ulceration (typically proximal to the medial malleolus, adjacent to the long saphenous vein); and surgical scars (these can be difficult to see sometimes).

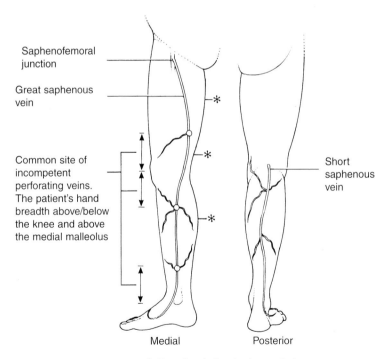

Saphenofemoral junction

Great saphenous vein

Common site of incompetent perforating veins. The patient's hand breadth above/below the knee and above the medial malleolus

Short saphenous vein

Medial   Posterior

* Tourniquet sites to demonstrate presence of incompetent perforators

Fig. 10.1 Varicose veins

Varicose ulcers should be differentiated from arteriopathic, neuro-pathic, diabetic, vasculitic (particularly rheumatoid), infective (e.g. syphilitic) and malignant ulcers. Arterial ulcers are usually sited on the lateral border of the lower limb, proximal to the lateral malleolus (i.e. furthest from the dorsalis pedis and posterior tibial arteries). (see Table 10.1)

Use palpation to confirm what you suspect from inspection. Remember to check both sides, as the limbs may have a different distribution of varicose veins. With the patient still standing, start proximally and confirm that the soft (bluish) reducible swelling over the saphenofemoral junction (just medial to the femoral artery if you are in any doubt), which has a fluid thrill when the patient coughs and empties on direct pressure, is a saphenous varix. Palpate the soft, but firm, varicose veins. You may be able to feel defects in the fascia – one (a patient's) hand-breadth proximal to the knee joint, one distal to the knee joint and one proximal to

Table 10.1	Common lower limb ulcers			
	Venous	Ischaemic	Trophic	Malignant
Site	Lower calf, typically superior to medial malleolus	Dorsum of foot over pressure points	Pressure points i.e. over metatarsals	May relate to venous ulcer or other scars
Associated conditions	Varicose veins Previous DVTs	Atherosclerosis Loss of peripheral pulses	Diabetic neuropathy Peripheral vascular disease Rheumatoid disease	Bowen's disease
Edge of ulcer	Shelving	Shelving	'Punched out' Deep	'Heaped' or everted
Base of ulcer	Frequently moist slough	Slough with poor granulation	Often dry eschar but may extend to bone	Frequently moist slough
Surrounding skin	Varicose eczema Liposclerosis	Thin and atrophic	May be normal	Dependent upon predisposing conditions

the medial malleolus. These may represent the sites of incompetent perforators from the deep to the superficial systems.

Percuss the column of blood in the great saphenous vein with one hand, while feeling with the other further proximally.

Trendelenburg's test   To determine the level of incompetent perforators (see Fig. 10.1):

1. Lie the patient on a couch, elevate the lower limb and empty the varicose veins.
2. Tighten a tourniquet around the upper thigh, hold the tourniquet in position, and ask the patient to stand.
3. If saphenofemoral incompetence is the sole cause of the varicosities, the varicose veins will not fill until you release the tourniquet 5 seconds later (when the veins fill rapidly). If the veins fill before the tourniquet is released, then there are other incompetent (perforator) veins distally.
4. Repeat the process – lie the patient down; empty the veins; apply the tourniquet distal to the site of the potentially incompetent perforator; stand the patient up; and look for varicosity filling before the tourniquet is released.
5. Continue until all the perforators are identified.

Remember to feel for the peripheral arterial pulses if there is an ulcer: it could be an ischaemic ulcer, even if the patient has varicose veins.

Investigation

In addition to the basic investigations for the assessment of a patient's fitness for anaesthesia (blood biochemistry and haematology, ECG, and chest radiology where appropriate), further investigation of the varicose veins is advisable if they are recurrent (to identify the incompetent perforators) or if there is a previous history of DVT (deep venous thrombosis) or lower limb trauma, to ensure that there is an intact deep venous system.

Doppler scanning for venous blood flow through incompetent valves (i.e. from the high-pressure deep venous system to the low-pressure superficial veins) can be used to identify the incompetent perforator veins, which may be sited at the classical positions (see Fig. 10.1). Alternatively, ascending venography can be used to map out the venous anatomy of the lower limb in complicated cases, particularly if the integrity of the deep venous system is in doubt (e.g. following a previous deep venous thrombosis).

Management

Conservative measures include the use of graduated compression stockings. Medical treatment does not have a role, but there are several surgical options. These range from injection sclerotherapy (for small veins distal to the knee), laser therapy (for small venous flares) and local ligation under local anaesthetic, to the standard high tie (saphenofemoral junction ligation) and the multiple ligation or avulsion of more distal vessels – to which may be added the stripping-out of the great saphenous vein from the groin to just distal to the knee, to reduce the chance of recurrence.

The swollen limb[†]

A swollen limb may be upper or lower, unilateral or bilateral, and due to general or localized problems. General problems causing bilateral lower limb swelling include cardiovascular causes (e.g. cardiac failure), renal causes (e.g. nephrotic syndrome) and low-protein states (e.g. hypoalbuminaemia). Local problems (which may cause unilateral or bilateral swelling of the lower limb) can be categorized as venous obstruction (e.g. DVT), lymphatic obstruction or intra-abdominal or intrathoracic obstruction of the venous or lymphatic systems. Lower limb swelling is more common in surgical finals than is upper limb swelling, which is comparatively rare except in patients with treated breast cancer.

Deep venous thrombosis[†]

Key points

- Predisposing factors: immobility
- 7–10 days post-operatively
- Symptoms of pulmonary embolism

History

Ask how long the limb has been swollen, in what circumstances the swelling was first noted, and whether the limb is painful. The recent history should include questions about recent surgery (particularly hip, knee or intra-abdominal surgery), immobility, trauma to the limb or pelvis, malignancy and medications (particularly the oral contraceptive pill and oestrogen-containing preparations). A past history of deep venous thrombosis or pulmonary embolism is important. The patient may tell you what medications he or she has been or is taking (heparin? warfarin?). Ask about respiratory symptoms, thinking of pulmonary embolism, particularly sharp (pleuritic) chest pain on inspiration, haemoptysis or breathlessness. Typically, deep venous thrombosis becomes clinically apparent a few days postoperatively and pulmonary embolism appears 7–10 days postoperatively.

Long-term sequelae of DVT may be the development of 'post-thrombotic syndrome', characterized by chronic limb swelling, dilated veins, varicose eczema and ulceration.

Examination

Expose the lower limbs up to the groin, with the patient lying comfortably on a bed or couch. Is there a pump administering heparin (the name of the drug should be written on the syringe or bag)? Look at the distribution of the swelling: is it unilateral or bilateral, and how far proximally does it extend up each limb? For a more objective test, measure the circumference of the calf and that of the thigh, and compare them with those of the opposite side. Are the classical signs of a red, swollen limb with shiny skin and visible superficial veins apparent (not all features may be present)?

Having asked the patient whether the limb is tender (and if so, where the tenderness is), gently compare the temperature of the two limbs using the dorsum of your fingers. With gentle pressure, elicit pitting oedema. Homan's sign (dorsiflexion of the ankle to elicit calf pain) is a very nonspecific sign of DVT, and many clinicians would not encourage you to use it. Gentle palpation of the calf and over the adductor canal may elicit discomfort in a patient with DVT.

You should ask to go on to examine the respiratory system if you suspect a pulmonary embolus (listen particularly for a localized pleural rub over the infarcted lung).

Percussion or auscultation of the limb is not helpful.

Investigation

Because the symptoms and signs of a deep venous thrombosis or pulmonary embolus are nonspecific, a high index of clinical suspicion, based on the patient's history, may be all that you have to suggest the diagnosis. The Radiology and Medical Physics Departments perform the key investigations.

Doppler scanning, to detect blood flow in the deep veins of the lower limb, is noninvasive but less specific than ascending venography, which can outline the veins containing thrombus. Techniques using radioisotopes to detect thrombus have a vogue in some centres.

In the case of pulmonary embolism, the radiological features on a chest film may be nonspecific, simply showing small segmental defects. Similarly, the ECG appearances of changes in the S wave in lead I, and changes in the Q and T waves in lead III, are not diagnostic. However, a perfusion scan may show segmental defects and when combined with a ventilation scan (to show ventilation/perfusion mismatch) will indicate the probability (low, medium or high) that pulmonary embolism has occurred. Pulmonary angiography, although rarely performed, is the definitive investigation. Increasing use of spiral CT scanning may mean that this soon becomes the investigation of choice.

Management

Conservative measures for the prevention of deep venous thrombosis include the use of graduated compression stockings, pneumatic compression boots and early postoperative mobility. Medical prevention may include the use of subcutaneous injections of heparin.

Formal treatment of deep venous thrombosis is aimed at preventing the extension or detachment of a segment of thrombus, and hence pulmonary embolism. Treatment comprises intravenous heparin infusion (some authorities recommend subcutaneous heparin injection as an alternative) with conversion to oral warfarin after 3 days, to maintain a therapeutic level of anticoagulation for 3–6 months. A vena caval filter may be indicated for patients with recurrent thromboembolism (from the lower limb or pelvic veins) despite adequate anticoagulation.

Lymphatic disease[†]

Lymphoedema may be primary (failure of the lymphatics to develop – more likely in the lower limbs than the upper limbs, and comparatively rare) or secondary (due to mechanical obstruction of the lymphatics, as a result of a disease process or of surgical or radiotherapy treatment).

A lymphoedematous limb is particularly prone to sepsis, and so a patient has to be aware of the potential problems (e.g. cellulitis and lymphangitis) that may arise from even quite minor abrasions. Rarely, a sarcoma may develop in the axilla of a lymphoedematous limb.

History

Patients in surgical finals with lymphoedema are likely to have had a tumour or treatment for a cancer involving the surgical excision of regional nodes, or radiotherapy to the regional nodes. The most likely cause of upper limb oedema is breast cancer (because of tumour infiltration, or surgery or radiotherapy to the axilla). In the case of the lower limb, intra-abdominal causes (particularly tumours) are likely for bilateral oedema (if one excludes cardiovascular disease and hypoproteinaemia), and one likely cause of unilateral lymphoedema is dissection of groin nodes (e.g. in melanoma).

In a long case, make sure that you ascertain a clear sequence of events and treatments: often the patient will be quite helpful.

Examination

With the limb in question and the contralateral limb exposed, look for surgical scars or signs of radiotherapy and compare the two sides. In the case of the upper limb, remember to inspect the chest wall for signs of treated or advanced breast cancer. Look to see whether the patient is wearing a compression stocking or armlet, or whether this is nearby. A graduated compression boot or sleeve, which uses a pump, may also be nearby.

Prior to palpation, ask whether the limb is tender or sore anywhere. Avoid tender areas. Gentle palpation will distinguish between a pitting oedema and a chronic, woody, non-pitting oedema.

Percussion or auscultation is not likely to be helpful.

Investigation

The investigation of lymphoedema should be aimed at discovering the cause. This may be self-evident from the history and inspection (e.g. a patient with breast cancer treated by mastectomy, axillary node clearance and radiotherapy).

Treatment

If a tumour is causing obstruction of the lymphatics, radiotherapy may result in reduction of the lymphoedema. However, upper limb lymphoedema is usually secondary to radiotherapy or surgery (or both) in the axilla and will rarely improve with (further) radiotherapy, so treatment is aimed at trying to minimize the swelling by using an arm-stocking and an intermittent pneumatic compression armlet.

Key questions

1. What are the features of claudication?
2. What are the signs of arterial insufficiency of the lower limb in:
   - acute ischaemia?
   - chronic ischaemia?
3. How does the presentation of acute limb ischaemia differ from that of chronic arterial occlusion?
4. How would you investigate a patient with claudication?
5. What is the significance of rest pain in a patient with peripheral vascular disease, and how should this be managed?
6. What is the difference between wet gangrene and dry gangrene?
7. Are the following true or false?
   - Arteriovenous malformations may cause excessive limb growth
   - The brachial artery is in danger from supracondylar humeral fractures
8. What are the predisposing factors for varicose veins?
9. How would you examine a patient with varicose veins?
10. How would you investigate and treat a patient with DVT (deep venous thrombosis)?
11. What are the long-term sequelae of DVT?
12. What are the likely causes and complications of unilateral upper limb oedema?

11

Limbs (locomotor) and back

Patients with orthopaedic problems make good short cases from the examiners' point of view, as they test your knowledge of basic anatomy, your clinical examination and whether you have attended the orthopaedic parts of your clinical attachments. A long case patient may have multiple medical problems as well as the principal condition (e.g. rheumatoid arthritis with cardiovascular and renal disease), which you may need to consider. Follow the now familiar scheme of history and examination. The scheme of inspection, palpation, percussion and auscultation is modified for orthopaedic patients to:

- look
- feel
- move.

THE LIMBS

HISTORY

The key areas to ask about include a history of trauma, analgesia and other medications, and orthopaedic operations. Questions should also be asked about the everyday functioning of the patient (e.g. stiffness, mobility, functional grip, walking, pain). Additional medical problems can, as for patients with vascular disease, influence the management options available.

EXAMINATION

Look

Begin your inspection with observation of the patient's posture and, if you are permitted to watch the patient walk (unusual in a surgical exam), his or her gait. Look for kyphosis, scoliosis, obvious deformities of the limbs (perhaps from a stroke resulting in upper and lower limb deficits) and facial paralysis.

Feel

Gently palpate visible lumps, contractures, joint line tenderness and effusions (particularly at the knee).

Move

Assess the active movement of joints, including the range of movement (ask the patient to flex or extend the joint), before you proceed to test passive movement. Once again, ensure that you are not causing pain.

Test for motor power, reflexes and sensation, particularly if you think there is likely to be an abnormality.

TYPICAL CASES

Fractures[†]

Key points

- Mechanism of injury
- Functional effects
- Related soft tissue injuries

You are very unlikely to see a patient with an acute fracture in your exam, but it is not uncommon for you to be faced with a patient with a treated fracture and to be examined on the initial and subsequent management of this patient. Remember that there may also be significant soft tissue injury. Of particular importance are injuries to adjacent neurovascular structures, and these must be looked for carefully at the time of injury.

History

Ask about how the fracture (defined as loss of bone continuity) occurred; the mechanism of the injury (e.g. falling onto an outstretched hand for a Colles' fracture); and whether there was a single injury or multiple trauma (perhaps in a road traffic accident). Was the fracture simple or compound (in which the skin or epithelium overlying the fracture is breached, increasing the risk of sepsis)? Ask about predisposing factors such as osteoporosis, previous injury, previous surgery and previous malignant disease (thinking particularly of bone metastases).

How was the fracture managed? Ask about the analgesia required; the method of anaesthesia; the method of reduction and fixation (manipulation and closed reduction, or open surgery – with or without wires, screws or prostheses); and whether antibiotics or antitetanus were given prophylactically.

Examination

Ensure that you have adequately exposed the limb bearing the fracture, acknowledging that this may be quite difficult if a plaster of Paris (or more modern substitute) is in place, and make sure that the patient is positioned comfortably.

Describe what you can see: this sounds obvious, but it is easy to forget to describe the presence of a plaster or an external fixation device, an obvious deformity, muscle wasting, skin discoloration, loss of skin, scars (surgical or traumatic) or swelling. Comment on whether a joint appears to be involved. Remember to compare the limb with the contralateral limb.

Ask if the limb is painful at any site. Feel the temperature of the injured limb, and feel for swelling, pitting oedema, bony discontinuity or protrusions. Feel whether a joint is likely to be involved.

Ask the patient to move the limb (active movement), to determine the range of movement compared with that of the contralateral limb, and the ease of movement. By passive movement of the limb, determine whether there is any abnormal movement (there is unlikely to be bony crepitus in an exam patient, but there may be malunion). Remember that a plaster may obstruct the full range of active or passive movement.

Investigation

Patients needing surgery, particularly the elderly or multiple-trauma patient, will require haematology, blood biochemistry, ECG and chest radiology, but the key investigation for a patient with a fracture is radiology. This must include two views, and must include the joint proximal to and the joint distal to the fracture. ,

Describe the fracture as far as you can, including:

- type and location of fracture (e.g. a simple/compound fracture of the mid-tibia)
- pattern of the fracture (e.g. transverse/spiral/comminuted (multiple fragments))
- the deformity (e.g. displacement/angulation/rotation)
- predisposing factors
- complicating factors.

Angulation should be described in terms of the direction in which the distal fragment is tilted (e.g. a Colles' fracture of the wrist, with radial and dorsal tilt).

Certain fractures (e.g. of the scaphoid) only really show up at a later date, on a radioisotope bone scan.

Treatment

The treatment of any fracture should aim to restore the continuity of the bone and return the patient to full mobility with the minimum of delay. However, fracture treatment may have to take second place in the multiply-injured patient, in whom immediate life-saving measures take precedence over the perhaps more dramatic fracture. Always remember that priority must be given to:

- A for Airway, with cervical spine control
- B for Breathing
- C for Circulation (fracture stabilization, with an external splint, may reduce blood loss).

Specific fracture treatment can be summarized as:

1. Initial splinting of the fracture and analgesia
2. Cleaning, and removal of devitalized tissue (debridement) if compound
3. Reduction of significant deformity

4. Maintenance of reduction until there is sound bony union
5. Intervention in response to any complicating factors, such as vascular impairment, if necessary
6. Full rehabilitation.

There are many different types of fracture and you are unlikely to be asked details about the management of specific individual fractures. Fracture treatment can range from analgesia and a sling (e.g. clavicle), through to a plaster cast (Colles'), internal fixation (femur), external fixation (tibia), hemiarthroplasty (hip) or total joint replacement (hip). The following fractures are sometimes encountered in surgical finals, and illustrate the general principles of fracture management.

Colles' fracture[†]

Site – within 2.5 cm of the wrist
Cause – fall on the outstretched hand
Associated features – osteoporosis (common in elderly women)
Deformity – dorsal and radial displacement
         – dorsal tilt of distal fragment
Treatment – manipulation if >10° of angulation
         – plaster from metacarpal phalangeal joint to below elbow
Complications – stiffness at wrist
              – possibility of frozen shoulder due to enforced immobility of upper limb
              – persisting deformity (e.g. malunion)
              – carpal tunnel syndrome
              – Sudeck's atrophy.

Fractured neck of femur[†]

Site – intracapsular (e.g. subcapital, transcervical)/extracapsular (e.g. intertrochanteric, subtrochanteric)
Cause – e.g. even apparently minor fall in elderly women
Associated features – this is generally a fracture associated with osteoporosis in the elderly
Deformity – clinically the limb is shortened and externally rotated
Treatment – usually by internal fixation: this allows early mobilization and minimizes the risk of non-union

Complications – patients with these fractures are frequently elderly and susceptible to hypostatic pneumonia, bed sores, urinary infections, deep venous thrombosis, pulmonary embolus and muscle wasting if left immobile for a long time. Avascular necrosis of the femoral head is more likely with intracapsular fractures. Non-union may occur if the diagnosis is delayed, or fixation is inadequate.

Rheumatoid arthritis*

Key points

- Multiple joints symmetrically affected
- Effects on function
- Systemic manifestations

There are several aspects of rheumatoid arthritis which you may encounter in either surgical or medical finals. In surgery, you are most likely to be asked to comment on a patient's hands, a rheumatoid nodule or a specific joint as a short case. Occasionally you may encounter a patient with rheumatoid arthritis in your long case, in which event you will have to determine: the features of the arthropathy; systemic features of the disease; treatment already received; planned future management; and other (unrelated) conditions.

Rheumatoid arthritis is usually symmetrical, typically affecting the following joints in middle-aged women: metacarpophalangeal (MCP), proximal interphalangeal (PIP), wrist, elbow, hip, knee, ankle, metatarsophalangeal and cervical.

History

Ask about the features of the arthropathy: the joints affected, the time-scale of the disease, the severity of acute exacerbations and the baseline disease. Typically patients will complain of pain and/or loss of function. With loss of function in particular you should determine what impact this has on your patient's life-style, i.e. can the patient dress him- or herself and cope with day-to-day activities? Does he or she use adapted or special appliances?

Many treatments for rheumatoid arthritis have significant side effects, so ask both what treatments have been prescribed previously and what is currently being used. Ask about drug treatments and their side effects, e.g. non-steroidal anti-inflammatory drugs and dyspepsia; steroids and metabolic disturbances, dyspepsia and weight gain. This being surgical finals, be sure to document any operations that have already been performed.

Rheumatoid arthritis is a systemic autoimmune disease, and you should ask the patient about any extra-articular symptoms suggestive of Sjögren's syndrome (dry eyes and mouth, parotid swelling); vasculitis (unusual rashes or leg ulcers); anaemia; renal failure; amyloidosis; sensory neuropathy; or Felty's syndrome (rheumatoid arthritis, splenomegaly, and pancytopenia).

Examination

Whether you are approaching a patient for the long case or a short case, take a moment to look for a walking stick, walking frame or wheelchair.

Examination should start with observation of the patient's gait, although in a short case when you ask if you can stand the patient up and see him or her walk, this may be considered unnecessary by the examiner. On inspection of the exposed hands and forearms (note how the patient undresses), look to see how the patient moves the hands. Are they obviously painful or limited in movement? Ask the patient to show you the palms and then the dorsa of the hands. Look for surgical scars (e.g. from synovectomy; hip, knee and digital joint replacements; joint stabilization) and for rheumatoid nodules. Rheumatoid nodules are subcutaneous masses, usually on the forearm or over the olecranon, that are typical of rheumatoid arthritis. You should treat the nodules like any other lumps you are asked to examine: describe their size, position, shape, degree of fixation (they will be mobile) and consistency (soft), and additional features (in this case the presence of rheumatoid arthritis). Look at the skin (is it atrophic? is there erythema or bruising?) and look for signs of muscle wasting. The typical deformity in rheumatoid arthritis of the hands is of ulnar deviation and subluxation at the metacarpophalangeal joints. An acute exacerbation will be painful, and there may be swelling and erythema of the affected joints. Rheumatoid arthritis tends to affect the MCP and PIP joints rather than the DIP (distal interphalangeal) joints, which are more likely to be affected by osteoarthritis. Look for specific deformities (see Fig. 11.1), particularly the boutonnière and swan neck deformities of the fingers, and the Z deformity of the thumb.

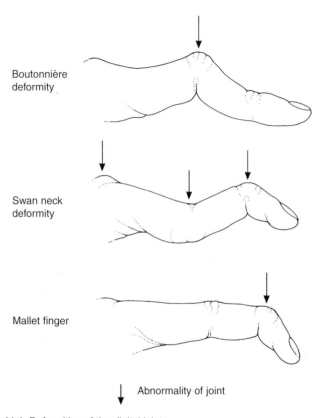

Boutonnière deformity

Swan neck deformity

Mallet finger

↓ Abnormality of joint

Fig. 11.1 Deformities of the digital joints

Ask if there are any tender areas, and avoid palpating these if possible. Gently feel the temperature of the skin overlying the joints, and palpate the soft tissue around the joint and the nodules.

Ask the patient to demonstrate the range of active movement that they have. Test the range of passive movement and then the power of each limb. Often, rheumatoid hands are used to test you in the exam, so remember to test pinch grip and the interossei (see p. 179).

Investigation

Since rheumatoid arthritis may have multiple systemic manifestations, it is not surprising that a full blood count may show anaemia (or pancytopenia in Felty's syndrome) and that the ESR may be very high in active disease. Blood biochemistry may provide evidence of renal compromise (due to the disease itself or secondary to drug therapy).

Following your examination, you may be asked to comment on limb or cervical radiographs. There is a progression of findings as the disease process develops: narrowing of the joint space; osteoporosis; lytic lesions in the periarticular bone; deformity due to subluxation of the joint; and finally, secondary osteoarthritis. In the cervical spine laxity of the atlanto-axial ligaments and odontoid peg may head to cord compression and so cervical spine radiographs are essential prior to any general anaesthetics.

Management

Conservative management of rheumatoid arthritis includes physiotherapy and splintage to avoid deformity, together with drug therapy. Surgery may have a role to remove thickened, inflamed synovium (synovectomy), stabilize unstable joints (arthrodesis), relieve disability and improve function in a destroyed joint (arthroplasty) and treat related soft tissue lesions such as tendon repairs and nerve decompressions.

Osteoarthritis

Whereas rheumatoid arthritis is an autoimmune disease, involving synovial joints, osteoarthritis can be regarded as being due to wear and tear and so is more common in the weight-bearing joints, particularly the hips and knees. Anything that increases the stress on a joint may predispose to osteoarthritis, particularly: obesity; previous fracture with persisting deformity; fracture through a joint; congenital deformities; rheumatoid arthritis; hard manual labour (e.g. miners); and sport.

Osteoarthritis of the hip[†]

Key points

- Pain and effects on daily activity
- Walking aids
- Limb shortening, deformities, muscle wasting
- Range of movement
- Muscle power

History

Ask the patient about pain in the hip, which is often worse on weight bearing, particularly on rising, but may wake the patient at night, when the muscles are relaxed. You should also ask about mobility and about any loss of function – particularly, how this interferes with the patient's life-style and the use of any appliances at home. Find out about any predisposing factors, such as previous injuries, slipped epiphysis in adolescence, or use of steroids (e.g. thinking of avascular necrosis of the femoral head).

Examination

Examination of the hip should start with observation of the patient's gait. In practice, in an exam situation this is probably best left until the end of the examination – at the beginning, the patient will probably be on a couch awaiting your attention. Ask if you can stand the patient up and see him or her walking, explaining that you will be looking for the typical antalgic gait associated with a painful hip. Nine times out of ten your examiner will say this is not necessary. Check that the patient is lying comfortably (with one pillow), wearing the minimum of clothing from the waist down to preserve modesty but not hinder inspection or further examination. Ensure that the anterior superior iliac spines are level.

Look to see whether there is a walking stick or walking frame next to the patient. If there is, ask the patient whether he or she uses it. (This checks that it belongs to the patient and makes the examiner, if present, aware that you have spotted it.)

Start by assessing the resting position of the lower limb for shortening, rotation or flexion contractures; look for any scars from previous surgery; and comment on any muscle wasting (most marked in the quadriceps and gluteal muscles). In osteoarthritis of the hip, apparent shortening of the lower limb can be detected by measuring the distance from the anterior superior iliac spine to the medial malleolus on each side. Measuring from the anterior superior iliac spine to the greater trochanter will demonstrate whether any difference is due to shortening of the hip joint. Apparent shortening, due to flexion deformities and adduction, will be evident on measuring from the umbilicus to each medial malleolus. A fixed flexion deformity may be evident if, in the resting position, the patient's thigh is not in contact with the examination couch – this can be confirmed using Thomas' test (see below). At rest, external rotation of the lower limb (detected most easily by examining the position of the foot at rest) may be evident.

Palpation of the hip joint itself is difficult. Ask if there is any tenderness, then feel for increased temperature and gently palpate the hip.

Test active movement: ask the patient to flex then extend the hip; to adduct then abduct the lower limb; and to internally then externally rotate the hip. You need to give precise instructions, and beware of the patient cheating.

Passive movement will allow you to fully assess a fixed flexion deformity. Use Thomas' test: flex the contralateral hip fully (to flatten out the lumbar lordosis) – any flexion at the hip under scrutiny is due to a fixed flexion deformity in the hip.

Next, passively adduct then abduct the lower limb. Abduction and adduction should be tested with the pelvis fixed in a stationary position. With the patient lying on their back, ask them to dangle the contralateral leg over the side of the bed. Now place one hand over a line between the two anterior superior iliac spines and abduct the leg from the midline. When there is tilting of the pelvis (detected by your hand across the two anterior superior spines), the limit of abduction at the hip has been reached. Note that further abduction is possible by tilting the pelvis – hence the fixing of the pelvis during testing.

Then passively rotate the hip internally then externally, noting the range of movement and whether there is any pain on movement. Internal and external rotation should be tested with the hip and knee both flexed to 90°, to test true rotation at the hip.

Remember that movement may be limited by pain, and if the patient is sore after a certain range of movement do not attempt to move the leg even more.

Compare the range of movement in the two hip joints. Ideally a goniometer should be used to measure the range of movement in each direction for each hip. For each aspect of movement (flexion, extension, etc.), test power using the following grading system:

0 – no movement
1 – visible muscle contraction, no joint movement
2 – joint movement when gravity eliminated
3 – movement overcomes gravity
4– movement overcomes gravity and resistance
5– normal power.

Investigation

After the history and examination, you will often be shown the patient's radiographs. Hopefully the patient will have a relatively normal contralateral hip with which to compare the abnormal one, but this is by no means certain. As in rheumatoid disease, there is a progression of changes in osteoarthritis as follows: loss of joint space; osteosclerosis in the periarticular bone; cyst and osteophyte formation in the bone adjacent to the joint; and finally, collapse of the femoral head and the acetabular roof.

Management

Initial conservative management will include advice on weight loss, the use of a walking stick and non-steroidal anti-inflammatary drugs. As, pain and disability increase, there is a growing indication for total hip replacement which has the twin benefits of restoring function and reducing pain. Occasionally an intertrochanteric osteotomy may be utilized to shift the stresses placed on an arthritic hip but this is far less common than a total hip replacement.

Osteoarthritis of the knee[†]

Key points

- Pain and functional effects on daily activity
- Deformities, effusions and muscle wasting
- range of movement

History

Ask the patient about pain and stiffness in the knee joint and about how their life-style is affected. The patient may have noticed swelling or occasional locking of the knee (commonly associated with cartilage tears, but sometimes due to loose bodies). You should also ask about any predisposing causes of the arthritis, particularly trauma, sporting activities and previous orthopaedic operations. Although difficulty with stairs may be more commonly a feature of ligamentous injury (particularly of the cruciates) than of osteoarthritis, you should ask about walking up and down stairs: is there any apprehension, or sense of the knee being about to 'give way'?

Examination

Many of the steps in the examination of the osteoarthritic knee, or any other problematic knee, are similar to those in the examination of the hip. Expose the entirety of both lower limbs.

Inspect the whole leg, and then the knee. Are there any scars? Does it appear swollen? Is there any obvious deformity of the joint (valgus or varus)? Is there any muscle wasting, particularly of vastus medialis? Ideally, you should see the patient walk, to assess the gait, and watch the patient walk up and down stairs.

Before you touch the limb, ask if it is tender anywhere. Use the dorsa of your fingers to check the temperature of the knee, and compare it to that of the other side. Measure the circumference of the left and right thighs at the same distance (10 cm) proximal to the knee joint, to confirm any subjective impression of muscle wasting. With the knee flexed at 30–45°, palpate the patella and around its margins, then feel the lower femur, the tibia and the head of the fibula: comment on any tenderness or abnormal bony projections (most likely to be osteophytes). Remember to palpate along the medial and lateral cartilages, and over the origin and insertion of the collateral ligaments and the popliteal fossa.

Test for an effusion. Place one hand on the thigh and empty out the suprapatellar bursa. With that hand kept in place, gently compress the inner aspect of the knee at the hollow behind the patella, and as you do this watch the other side of the knee to see if there is any bulging (suggesting fluid). If you are unsure, repeat the procedure but stroke the outer aspect as you watch the inner aspect. A patellar tap is a good method of detecting a moderate or large effusion: empty the suprapatellar bursa, then use your other hand to demonstrate a springy tap by pressing sharply on the patella.

The movements of the knee are flexion and extension, with some rotation to lock the knee at the extreme of extension. As always, test active movements before progressing to passive movements. Comment on the range of movement and power (graded 0 to 5 – see p. 169) of the muscle groups.

Although it is unlikely to be useful in examination of the osteoarthritic knee, in other circumstances you may wish to test for any ligamentous laxity (medial and lateral collateral ligaments) and for anterior or posterior cruciate tears. To examine for collateral ligament laxity: with the lower limb almost fully extended (but the knee not locked), push one hand against the medial side of the knee to test for lateral collateral ligament laxity and vice versa. To examine for cruciate disruption (which may only be evident in the presence of collateral ligament disruption): flex the knee to 90°, fix the foot and, with the hamstring muscles relaxed, use two hands placed behind the upper tibia to test for the anterior drawer sign (anterior cruciate disruption) by attempting to pull the tibia towards you. Then, by pushing the tibia away from you, test for posterior cruciate laxity.

You are unlikely to be asked to perform the apprehension test (for patellar instability) or the McMurray test (for a torn meniscus) in surgical finals.

Investigation

After your examination of the knee, ask to inspect radiographs of the knee joint. The radiological signs of osteoarthritis of the knee are similar to those of osteoarthritis of the hip: narrowed joint space; osteosclerosis; cyst and osteophyte formation.

Management

As for osteoarthritis of the hip, initial medical management includes NSAIDs, and life-style changes. Total knee replacement may be required as the joint becomes increasingly arthritic.

Peripheral nerve lesions*

Key points

- Knowledge of the site of injury and of the sensory and motor distributions of a nerve will allow you to predict the functional effects

These are much beloved by examiners as short cases – it gives them a chance to observe you examining, and also an opportunity to test your long-forgotten knowledge of anatomy. Peripheral nerve lesions are more likely to appear in a surgical exam than are general neuropathies (e.g. as seen in diabetics, alcoholics or as side effects of drugs, and in patients with primary neurological diseases). It is important in surgical finals to know the sensory distribution and motor function of the major peripheral nerves. Contrast these with the sensory distribution of the nerve roots and the muscles supplied by them: it can all become quite complex. Figure 11.2 shows a diagrammatical way of remembering some of the key points.

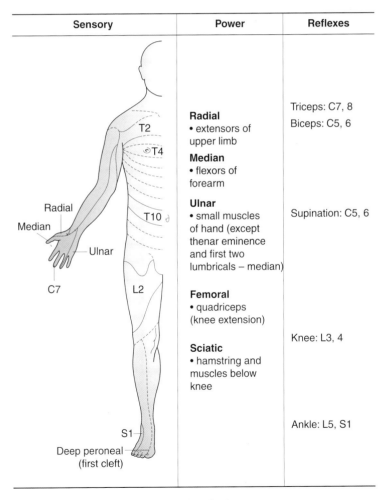

Sensory	Power	Reflexes
	Radial • extensors of upper limb **Median** • flexors of forearm **Ulnar** • small muscles of hand (except thenar eminence and first two lumbricals – median) **Femoral** • quadriceps (knee extension) **Sciatic** • hamstring and muscles below knee	Triceps: C7, 8 Biceps: C5, 6 Supination: C5, 6 Knee: L3, 4 Ankle: L5, S1

Fig. 11.2 Sensory and motor nerve aide-mémoire

History

Ask about any history of trauma, the distribution of pain or paraesthesia, and any weakness. Enquire about the functional use of the limb in question, both in everyday life and at work. Ask whether any surgery (e.g. nerve repair, release of contractures, tendon transfer) has been performed.

Examination

With the limb under examination and the contralateral limb exposed, inspect for any scars (self-inflicted trauma is a common cause of median nerve damage) and muscle wasting. Is the limb held in a particular position, as in Erb's palsy?

Test the power of the muscle groups in the limb you are examining, and make comparisons with the contralateral limb. If you suspect a peripheral nerve lesion, pay particular attention to the muscle group(s) supplied by that nerve.

Test for sensation. Use a blunted (but unused) phlebotomy needle to test for pinprick sensation, then cotton wool to test for light touch. The other components of sensation (vibration and temperature) are perhaps more relevant in medical finals. Having established that there is sensory loss, map out the distribution.

Test for limb reflexes using a tendon hammer.

Try to work out whether the neurological deficit suggests a nerve root problem or a peripheral nerve lesion. Fortunately, only a few of the many possible nerve lesions are commonly encountered in exams. Some of these are described below.

Upper brachial plexus lesion[§]

The condition known as Erb's palsy results from injury to one or more cervical nerve roots, often C5/C6.

Cause – obstetric trauma, fall on tip of shoulder
Position – arm held internally rotated, forearm pronated
Sensory deficit – outer aspect of the arm
Motor deficit – abduction at the shoulder, flexion at the elbow
Treatment – await recovery; physiotherapy for passive joint movements. Arthrodesis at the shoulder and elbow may be considered.

Lower brachial plexus lesion[†]

The condition known as Klumpke's palsy typically involves damage to the roots of C8/T1.

Cause – usually secondary to trauma (e.g. stretching injury of a motorcyclist dragged along the ground). Rarely, due to a Pancoast's tumour, birth trauma, or a cervical rib

Position – clawhand (hyperextension of the metacarpophalangeal joints); more pronounced on the ulnar side of the hand

Sensory deficit – inner aspect of forearm; three and a half fingers on the ulnar side of the hand

Motor deficit – weakened flexion and ulnar deviation at the wrist; loss of adduction and abduction of the fingers

Treatment – await recovery; physiotherapy for passive joint movements. Prognosis is less favourable than with Erb's palsy.

Radial nerve lesion[†]

Cause – in the axilla: fractures/dislocations of the humeral head; crutches without hand grips
– in the radial groove of the humerus: fractures of the humeral shaft; 'Saturday night paralysis' (due to drunken sleep with the arm over the back of a chair)

Position – drop wrist may be apparent

Sensory deficit – proximal division of the nerve leads to loss of sensation over the dorsum of the forearm and the dorsum of the first interosseus muscle

Motor deficit – extension of elbow and wrist (although the long extensors of the fingers are paralysed, the lumbricals can still extend the fingers); extension of the elbow may be saved when the nerve is divided distally

Treatment – initially, expectant; nerve suture may have a relatively good prognosis, as the radial nerve is predominantly motor.

Median nerve lesion[†]

See also the section on carpal tunnel syndrome (below).

Cause – at the elbow: supracondylar humeral fracture

– at the wrist: lacerations, and occasionally a Colles'
fracture; compression due to carpal tunnel syndrome

Position – Simian hand (due to wasting of the thenar muscles)

Sensory deficit – anaesthesia over palmar aspects of thumb and
index and middle fingers

Motor deficit – division of the median nerve at the wrist leads to
loss of opposition of the thumb; in more proximal
lesions there is a weakness of flexion at the wrist,
and loss of flexion of the IP (interphalangeal)
joint of the thumb

Treatment – suture of the nerve is required if there is obvious
division, but the prognosis is poor as this is a mixed
motor and sensory nerve.

Ulnar nerve lesion*

Cause – at the elbow: fractures, entrapment in the region of the
medial epicondyle
– at the wrist: lacerations

Position – clawing of the little, ring and middle fingers due to
wasting of the small muscles of the hand

Sensory deficit – loss over the little finger and half of the ring
finger, anteriorly and posteriorly if the lesion is
above the wrist; lesions at the wrist lead only to
anterior loss of sensation

Motor deficit – loss of adduction and abduction of the fingers;
with proximal lesions, there is weakness of the
long flexors of the little and ring fingers

Treatment – transposition of the nerve at the elbow, if entrapped.

Sciatic nerve lesion§

Cause – posterior dislocation of hip, 'intramuscular' injections

Sensory deficit – total loss of sensation below the knee, except for
the inner aspect of the calf

Motor deficit – complete paralysis below the knee; foot drop;
paralysis of the hamstrings.

Lateral popliteal nerve lesion*

Cause – fractures of the upper end of the fibula; pressure from
plasters; inappropriate positioning on the theatre table

Sensory deficit – lateral border of the foot
Motor deficit – dorsiflexion of the foot and dorsiflexion of the
              great toe (foot drop)
Treatment – splinting of the foot in the position of function and
            awaiting recovery; alternatively, decompression over
            the head of the fibula may be required.

Carpal tunnel syndrome*

Key points

- Median nerve distribution of symptoms
- Pressure over carpal tunnel may reproduce symptoms

History

The presenting symptom of carpal tunnel syndrome is usually
pain or paraesthesia, worse at night, in the distribution of the
median nerve in the hand and typically in a middle-aged female.
Although usually idiopathic, it may occur in cardiac failure,
rheumatoid arthritis, pregnancy, hypothyroidism, acromegaly, or
as a complication of a Colle's fracture.

Examination

With the forearm and hand exposed on both sides, inspection may
reveal a scar over the flexor retinaculum on one side (hopefully the
asymptomatic, successfully operated-upon side!). Motor loss is
unusual. There may be loss of sensation over the palmar aspects of
the thumb, index and middle fingers. Pressure on or tapping the
carpal tunnel (Tinel's sign) may reproduce the symptoms.

Investigation

Although these findings are commonly quoted in textbooks, nerve
conduction studies are required to confirm the diagnosis.

Treatment

Treatment is by division of the flexor retinaculum at the wrist,
distal to the wrist crease.

Dupuytren's contracture*

Baron Guillaume Dupuytren gained much esteem for treating Napoleon Bonaparte's piles. However, it is a condensation of the palmar fascia that bears his name and Dupuytren's contractures are common short cases in final exams.

History

You should find out which hand is the dominant hand, and how the contracture interferes with the patient's day-to-day activities. Ask about predisposing causes such as liver disease or recurrent trauma to the palm, remembering that in most patients the contracture has no recognizable cause.

Examination

On inspection then palpation, look for a condensation of the palmar fascia into nodules and a band, which may be felt in the palm. As the disease evolves, the fingers (most commonly the little and ring fingers) are drawn into flexion. Thereafter, there is increasing flexion at the MCP and IP joints, resulting in joint contractures.

Treatment

Treatment is by excision of the fibrous tissue. Once there is marked deformity of a digit it is usually difficult to straighten it, and amputation may give the best functional result.

Bursa*

Bursae are, of course, normally present over bony prominences. There are also adventitious bursae, which are newly formed cysts in areas with repeated trauma – the most common is the bursa overlying the first metatarsal in hallux valgus (a bunion). You are most likely to encounter bursae in your short cases, and most commonly a chronic bursitis, occurring in an area subjected to repeated stress.

Hand examination*

Sometimes you will be asked to examine a patient's hands. Remember to look for: nail changes; clubbing; nicotine stains; Heberden's nodes (DIP); Bouchard's nodes (PIP); gout tophi (periarticular; also on toes, pinnae); rheumatoid changes; bruising; muscle wasting (usually due to old age, rheumatoid arthritis or cachexia); warts; palmar erythema; Dupuytren's contracture; trigger finger; wasted thenar muscles; T1 root lesion (all the small muscles of the hand are atrophic, with little sensory loss) compared with ulnar nerve palsy (thenar muscles supplied by the median nerve are spared; sensory loss of the ulnar border of the hand); tremor (fine tremor of anxiety, thyrotoxicosis; 'pill rolling' tremor of Parkinson's disease); function (grip: ask the patient to squeeze two of your fingers; thumb: test strength in opposition to other index finger; test for Froment's sign (grip paper with thumb/index finger); functional use: holding cup, spoon); sensory loss (index finger tip (median nerve); little finger tip (ulnar nerve); dorsum of first interosseus muscle (radial nerve)); and radial pulse.

Finger clubbing*

Finger clubbing is so common that it usually appears somewhere in finals. You are rarely asked to take a history, but remember the causes if you are. The causes are many, but are best remembered as 'no cause' (idiopathic, familial – the commonest category); gastrointestinal (e.g. inflammatory bowel disease such as Crohn's, ulcerative colitis; liver cirrhosis); pulmonary (e.g. bronchogenic carcinoma; chronic suppurative lung diseases like bronchiectasis; fibrosing alveolitis); and heart disease (e.g. congenital cyanotic heart disease; infective endocarditis).

Examination

On examination, look for the yellow/brown staining of nicotine. Inspect the nails of both hands, commenting on the shape of the nails and terminal phalanges and the nail bed angle (between the nail and the proximal skin).

Gently palpate the nail bed: support the patient's digit with your own two thumbs then, using your index fingers, elicit fluctuance of the nail bed. You will probably only need to demonstrate this on one digit before you are asked to list some causes of clubbing.

Trigger finger[†]

Trigger finger (or trigger thumb) is due to the flexor tendon of the affected digit catching on its sheath at the metocarpophalangeal joint. When the patient straightens the fingers, the affected digit will remain flexed and then suddenly flick out into the extended position. There may be a palpable (sometimes tender) nodule to feel where the tendon catches.

Mallet finger[§]

A mallet finger results from the rupture of the long extensor tendon where it inserts into the distal phalange, producing a typical deformity (see Fig. 11.1).

THE BACK

The back has been included in this chapter because patients with nerve root compression due to back problems may present with lower limb symptoms in surgical finals. In such a case you will be expected to differentiate between the compression of a nerve root and a specific peripheral nerve lesion. The most common presentation of pathology in the back is pain, usually in the lumbar region.

HISTORY

If you are presented with a patient with back problems, establish their age. Disc problems are most common in the age range 30–45 years, after which there is a progressive increase in the incidence of osteoarthritis. In older patients, metastatic carcinoma should be considered. Ask particularly about the onset, site, radiation, exacerbating factors, relieving factors and severity of any pain, which may lead you quickly to the diagnosis.

An acute disc prolapse will often occur when the patient has lifted something heavy or sneezed, and is associated with severe pain and 'locking' of the back. The pain may well shoot down the patient's leg in the distribution of L5 or S1 nerve roots (from the buttock to distal to the knee). Disc pain may have a more chronic onset and present first with nerve root irritation. Similarly, other causes of back pain may have an insidious onset (e.g. metastatic disease, osteoarthritis and spondylolisthesis). In addition to asking about back pain and radiation of the pain, find out about the impact of the symptoms on the patient's life-style. Ask particularly about the patient's work, and whether there is any question of industrial injury or compensation claims. You must not forget to enquire about related medical problems, such as osteoarthritis in other joints, the possibility of metastatic cancer (often lung, breast or prostate) or referred to the back from other sites, such as the pancreas. Finally remember that back pain may be a symptom of intra–abdominal pathology, i.e. an aortic aneurysm or a pancreatic carcinoma.

EXAMINATION

Your system for examining the back should follow the same pattern as that established for other orthopaedic problems:

- look
- feel
- move.

Following this, you should conduct a full neurological examination, looking for signs of nerve root compression.

Look

It is helpful to watch a patient's gait and examine the spinal curvature with the patient wearing a minimum of underclothes, so that you can observe movements of the spine. Look particularly for the typical 'half-shut knife' position of someone leaning forward with a partially flexed, painful back. There may be flattening of the normal lumbar lordosis due to erector spinae spasm, which if more marked on one side may lead to a scoliosis. Comment also on any visible 'steps' or marked kyphosis which may have resulted from vertebral collapse.

Feel

Ask whether the patient has any tenderness before you palpate the spine. Localized tenderness may occur over an area of pathology, and may identify the level of a lesion. Unfortunately, it will not differentiate between different types of lesion affecting the back, e.g. crush fractures, metastatic disease or disc problems. You may be able to feel a specific 'step' in cases of spondylolisthesis, or a localized kyphosis in a patient with vertebral collapse.

Move

Test for flexion and extension, but watch to see that the back is moving: a patient with ankylosing spondylitis, when asked to touch his toes, may bend forwards at the hips even though the back is completely fused. Lateral flexion to the left and to the right should be determined, again watching to ensure that this is not achieved by tilting the pelvis. Holding the pelvis steady, assess rotation to the left and to the right. Flexion, extension, lateral flexion and rotation can be tested for the cervical, thoracic and lumbar spine, recognizing that the range of each type of movement will be different in each part of the spine.

With the patient lying supine, perform the straight leg raise: with the knee fully extended, gently elevate the leg – there will be limitation of straight leg raising if there is nerve root irritation. Dorsiflexion of the foot or pressure over the popliteal fossa will exacerbate sciatic nerve pain radiating from the lumbar spine to distal to the knee. Movement at the hip may be free, and often there is a full range of hip flexion provided that the knee is flexed. The femoral stretch test (with the patient lying prone and the hip passively extended) is not very likely to be required of you in the exam.

Neurological examination

If you suspect vertebral collapse or a prolapsed disc it is essential to assess the patient's neurological status (see Fig.11.2). This will involve the assessment of:

- power (graded 0 to 5, see p. 169),
- sensation (to pinprick and touch as a basic minimum),
- reflexes (in the affected limbs),

and comparing the findings with your assessment of the contra-lateral limb.

TYPICAL CASES

Lumbar disc prolapse[†]

This is the commonest type of disc prolapse, and the one most likely to be encountered in exams.

History

Take a history as outlined above, asking particularly about the patient's job, the symptoms of pain (which should be differentiated from pain due to peripheral vascular disease), and the limitations they impose on everyday activities such as sitting and bending (e.g. putting on socks). Paraesthesia or numbness may also be symptoms of disc prolapse or nerve compression, and establishing which parts of the limb have altered sensation will often guide you to the nerve roots involved. Loss of control of the bladder or bowel are unlikely to be present in a patient used in surgical finals, but you should still ask about these symptoms, as they imply a surgical emergency. Ask what analgesia or other relieving tactics (such as lying on the floor) have been tried.

Examination

The patient with an acute disc prolapse will hold their back in a slightly flexed position, and you will see loss of the normal lordosis and marked erector spinae spasm.

It is likely that there will be tenderness over the relevant vertebral body, and also over the tense erector spinae muscles.

The most common disc prolapses are L4/L5 (catching the L5 nerve root) and L5/S1 (affecting the S1 nerve root). In both cases there is limitation of straight leg raising. Lesions affecting L5 will cause weakness of dorsiflexion of the ankle and of the great toe, and sensory loss over the dorsum of the foot. The ankle jerk will be present. In contrast, S1 lesions will result in loss of the ankle jerk, weakness of plantar flexion of the ankle and toes, and anaesthesia along the outer aspect of the foot. Rarely, prolapse of a higher disc may affect the L4 nerve root, resulting in weakness of the quadriceps and loss of the knee jerk reflex. In this case, stretching the femoral nerve is painful. This is done by asking the patient to lie on their front and gently extending the hip with the knee flexed.

Occasionally, a disc prolapse will protrude centrally, compressing the spinal cord. This will lead to bilateral symptoms, loss of anal sphincter control and bladder paresis. It is very unlikely that you will see such a patient in the exam, as this is a surgical emergency, but you may be asked about it. Cervical disc lesions are much less common than lumbar disc problems, and neurological sequelae are unusual because of the comparatively large vertebral foramen in the cervical region.

Investigation

The differential diagnosis of lumbar disc prolapse includes osteoarthritis, spondylolisthesis, metastatic tumours and primary and secondary spinal tumours. You should therefore ask for blood biochemistry including urea, electrolytes, calcium, phosphate, and prostate specific antigen (PSA – a marker of prostate cancer), and for the ESR.

A plain radiograph may not show any specific lesion, but may help to exclude part of the differential diagnosis. Prolapse of a disc through the end plate into the vertebral body may result in the radiological appearance of a Schmorl's node. Other radiological signs may include narrowing of disc spaces and secondary osteoarthritic changes. If surgery is contemplated, the level of the disc prolapse should be identified from a CT or MRI scan. If metastatic disease is suspected, but not demonstrated on plain radiographs, then a bone scan may be informative and may demonstrate the cause of the symptoms.

Management

The majority of disc prolapses will resolve with conservative measures: bed rest and certainly the avoidance of any heavy lifting or vigorous activity until the pain subsides. Analgesia and antispasmodics can give great relief. In cases which either fail to settle or recur, surgery should be considered. An absolute and urgent indication for surgery is the development of bladder paralysis from a central disc prolapse. Progressive muscle weakness would also indicate the need for decompression. Microdiscectomy or hemilaminectomy should be performed in order to remove the prolapsed disc material.

Secondary tumour deposits in the vertebrae[†]

These are relatively common compared with primary spinal tumours as a cause of back pain, and may cause vertebral collapse and cord compression.

History

The patient may give you a history of a previous carcinoma, or alternatively this may be the first sign of a carcinoma (particularly in the case of prostatic carcinoma or multiple myeloma). The presentation may simply be back pain, or alternatively progressive vertebral collapse may lead to neurological symptoms such as pain in the girdle region and progressive weakness (usually of the lower limbs).

Examination

There may be little to see and only localized tenderness on examination of the back. Alternatively, you may see signs of vertebral collapse, including kyphosis or scoliosis. If there is cord compression the patient, if mobile, will have a broad-based gait. There may be signs of increased muscle tone and a spastic paresis in the lower limbs (typical of an upper motor neurone paralysis). Remember to look also for signs of the primary tumour, the most common being breast, prostate, bronchus, kidney and thyroid.

Investigation

Investigations should be performed in order to determine the site of the primary tumour. With regard to the bony lesion, clinical biochemistry may show elevated calcium and phosphate together with elevated alkaline phosphatase, but these are nonspecific indicators of bone activity.

Plain radiographs may demonstrate either sclerotic lesions (particularly in prostatic carcinoma and breast cancer) or lytic lesions, but may also be normal in the case of early lesions. A bone scan using radioisotopes will show an area of increased uptake corresponding to metastatic bone lesions, but this finding is nonspecific and should only be regarded as showing metastatic tumour if associated with normal radiographs or typical lesions of bony secondaries (rather than benign changes such as those of arthritis).

If there are signs of cord compression, the level and extent of this should be delineated by means of a CT or MRI scan.

Management

Conservative measures (such as the use of a walking stick) and analgesia may provide considerable relief. Rehydration (if bone metastases have caused hypercalcaemia) and treatment of the hypercalcaemia with bisphosphonates can be very effective.

Treatment of the primary tumour may also be effective in the treatment of the bony disease (e.g. tamoxifen in breast cancer or orchidectomy (surgical or chemical) in prostatic cancer). Localized radiotherapy is often successful in the control of pain due to the tumour. In cases where there is cord compression, it may be necessary to consider surgical decompression: when there is vertebral collapse, this will involve initial stabilization of the spine.

Key questions

1. What is the basic examination scheme for orthopaedic patients?
2. How would you describe a fracture?
3. In general terms, how would you treat a patient with a fracture?
4. What is the typical deformity of a Colles' fracture, and how is this fracture caused?
5. Which systems may be involved in rheumatoid arthritis?
6. How would you examine the hip?
7. How would you classify muscle power?
8. What are the features of an ulnar nerve palsy?
9. What are the key features of: ·
   • Dupuytren's contracture?
   • finger clubbing?
10. How would you differentiate between a ganglion and a sebaceous cyst?
11. What features of disease might you see on a patient's hands?
12. What are the differences between the neurological findings in a lateral peroneal nerve lesion and a prolapse of the L5/S1 intervertebral disc?

13. Answer the following true or false:
    - Prolapsed cervical discs commonly cause neurological symptoms T
    - Lumbar disc prolapse is a condition of the elderly F
    - Carpal tunnel syndrome leads to wasting of the interosseous muscles F
    - The radial nerve is commonly damaged in Colles' fractures F
    - The sciatic nerve is in danger following dislocation of the hip T
    - Rheumatoid arthritis usually affects the DIP joints F
    - The ankle jerk reflex is absent in an L5/S1 disc prolapse T
    - Bony metastases may not be apparent on plain radiographs T

PART 3

MISCELLANEOUS

12

Other useful topics

There are some topics which can come up in the clinical parts or the oral parts of surgical finals, and are usually related to a patient whom you have been asked to examine.

TRAUMA AND RESUSCITATION

Injury can be described as blunt injury, penetrating (knife/firearms) injury or blast injury. The history will give hints as to the likely patterns of injury. Whatever the type of injury, the ABC of trauma resuscitation forms the basis of how to resuscitate a patient following trauma, in any emergency situation including surgical finals:

- A for Airway, with cervical spine control
- B for Breathing
- C for Circulation.

A. Clear and then maintain the airway (while keeping the cervical spine controlled in the case of trauma patients):

- clear obstruction of the airway by foreign bodies/tongue
- maintain the airway by chin lift/jaw thrust
- insert an oropharyngeal airway/cuffed endotracheal tube, or use cricoid needle/cricothyroidotomy if required.

B. Ensure the patient is breathing:

- assist breathing if necessary
- supply high-flow oxygen if necessary
- beware (tension) pneumothorax and flail segments.

C. Control bleeding and maintain circulating blood volume:

- control external bleeding with pressure

- control internal bleeding if possible (e.g. splint fractures)
- restore circulating blood volume (using crystalloids and matched (preferably) or blood group O Rhesus negative blood), via two large-bore venous cannulae (use pulse and urine output as measures of circulating blood volume).

D. Conduct survey from head to toe of fully exposed patient, including all orifices.

Head injury:

- prevent secondary brain injury due to hypoxia, hypercapnia, hypotension, intracranial bleeding
- beware extradural haematoma (usually due to injury of the middle meningeal vessels) – classically presents with a transient loss of consciousness, a lucid interval, then deterioration of the conscious level
- beware facial/mandibular fractures, causing airway impairment and/or blood loss.

Chest injury:

- beware tension pneumothorax/haemothorax
- beware rib fractures
- beware cardiac injury
- beware penetrating injuries.

Abdominal injury:

- beware occult intra-abdominal bleeding (a diagnostic peritoneal lavage may be needed)
- perform rectal examination
- test urine for blood
- catheterize if no urethral or perineal injury
- insert nasogastric tube.

Extremity injuries:

- splint injured limbs, to reduce pain and blood loss
- control bleeding from vascular injuries
- beware compartment syndrome
- clean, debride and explore wounds
- ensure antitetanus prophylaxis.

FLUID BALANCE/NUTRITION

Some patients in surgical finals may have a drip attached, or may be receiving parenteral nutrition.

Fluid/electrolyte balance

The topic of fluid and electrolyte balance can give you sleepless nights, trying to remember exact values and the many upset states that are possible in patients. The essential concept to remember is that what is lost must be replaced. Working out the types of fluid/electrolytes lost, and the sites of loss, gives you a clue to the patient's requirements.

A normal adult's basic daily needs are:

- sodium, 70–80 mmol (one 500 ml bag of 0.9% saline)
- potassium, 60 mmol (falling to 20 mmol first postoperatively day)
- water, 1000 ml (minimum).

The possible routes, and the corresponding extents, of fluid losses and gains are summarized in Table 12.1. Those represented by a '?' are highly variable.

Table 12.1   Fluid balance

Losses	ml/day	Gains	ml/day
Normal			
Urine	1500	Endogenous water	300
Insensible			
–breathing	700		
– sweat	200		
Faeces	200		
Possible			
Gastric (nasogastric tube/vomit)	2500	Oral	?
Bile duct (via T tube)	1500	Intravenous	?
Pancreatic	1000	IV additives	?
Small bowel fistula	3000	Central line	?
Diarrhoea	15 000		
Sequestration			
– to wound site	500		
– from drains	?		
– into chest cavity	?		
– peritoneum (ascites)	?		

Nutrition

The normal daily nutritional requirements of a 70 kg man are:

- 9–15 g nitrogen
- 2000–3000 kcal (including 200 kcal of non-protein energy per g of nitrogen, of which 60–80 kcal should be provided by fat)
- 2–3l fluid
- electrolytes (including 70 mmol sodium and 60 mmol potassium)
- trace elements, minerals and vitamins.

Nutrition can be given via the gastrointestinal tract (the enteral route – by mouth or by tube (nasogastric, nasoduodenal, gastrostomy or jejunostomy)), or intravenously as parenteral nutrition (via a peripheral or central vein).

Oral/enteral nutrition can be in the form of normal food, fluid feed or elemental diet. Complications of the enteral route include nausea, vomiting, bloating and diarrhoea, and wound problems at the insertion site of the feeding tube (in the case of gastrostomy/ jejunostomy).

Complications of parenteral nutrition include those of catheter insertion (e.g. haematoma, pneumothorax, air embolus); thrombophlebitis (especially with peripheral lines); cardiac dysrhythmias (due to the tip of the line); and infection (at the skin entry site, or of the catheter); infection may in turn result in septicaemia; and metabolic disturbance (e.g. hyperosmolar syndrome, electrolyte imbalance, abnormal liver function, deficiency syndromes).

PREOPERATIVE INVESTIGATIONS

Preparation of a patient for surgery is one of the commonest tasks for recently qualified doctors – hence it is often a topic in surgical finals.

Cardiac disease, respiratory conditions and fluid/electrolyte disturance (see above) are key areas. While some investigations may be considered essential in all patients undergoing general anaesthesia (e.g. haemoglobin), patients aged > 45 years and patients with symptoms of cardiorespiratory disease require more rigorous investigations selected from the following list:

Investigations:

- urinary testing for glucose in diabetics, proteins in renal disease
- haematology may show anaemia (microcytic/macrocytic) as an exacerbating factor in cardiorespiratory symptoms

- prothrombin time ration or international normalised ratio for control of warfarin
- biochemistry (ureas, sodium, potassium) may confirm electrolyte disturbances which can precipitate or worsen cardiac dysrhythmias
- arterial blood gas for arterial PO_2, CO_2 and acid/base balance may confirm the presence of hypoxia or hypercarbia and/or compensatory changes in metabolic or respiratory acidosis or alkalosis
- blood transfusion – group and save, cross match (number of units depends on likely extent of surgery)
- chest PA radiograph
- a 12 lead ECG may be used to assess cardiac rate and rhythm and signs of current or previous myocardial damage
- a treadmill/stress ECG and/or 24-hour monitoring tape may elicit signs of myocardial disease
- echocardiography can be used to examine the structure and function of the heart muscle, heart valves and blood flow
- spirometry may be used to measure the FEV1, FVC, FEV1/ FVC ratio and more complex measures of respiratory function.

ANALGESIA

Although this subject is covered fully in textbooks on anaesthesia, analgesia is a favourite topic when discussing postoperative patient management, perhaps as part of a long case. You should be able to discuss the following methods and their uses:

Local analgesia
- skin gel
  - local anaesthetic
  - non-steroidal anti-inflammatory
- injected local anaesthetic
  - lignocaine (short-acting)
  - bupivicaine (long-acting)
- regional nerve blockade
  - local nerves (just as at the dentist!)
  - regional caudal block
  - epidural

Systemic analgesia
- paracetamol
- non-steroidal anti-inflammatory
- opiate
  - dihydrocodeine
  - pethidine
  - morphine

The methods of delivery of analgesia include oral (tablet/ sublingual/liquid); per rectum (suppository); intermittent injections; infusion; and patient-controlled analgesia (PCA). Antiemetics can be added to these.

POSTOPERATIVE COMPLICATIONS

Postoperative complications, such as those listed, can occur following any operation.

Distant to site of surgery
- pulmonary atelectasis
- pneumonia
- fluid overload
- phlebitis
- DVT/pulmonary embolus
- urinary tract infection
- central line sepsis
- transfusion reactions
- renal failure
- pressure sores

At site of surgery
- haemorrhage
- nerve damage
- wound infection
- abscess
- ileus
- wound dehiscence
- anastomotic leakage
- fistula

DEEP VENOUS THROMBOSIS (DVT)

Development

DVT develops during/after 30% of surgical operations. The three main aetiological factors are venous stasis, enhanced coagulation and intimal damage (Virchow's triad). The many risk factors include: age of > 40 years; malignancy; obesity; abdominal surgery; hip/knee replacement surgery; previous DVT or embolus; and the oral contraceptive pill.

Prevention is assisted by: subcutaneous low-dose heparin started preoperatively (e.g. 5000u b.d.); graduated compression stockings; early mobilization; intermittent pneumatic compression boots intraoperatively and dextran 70.

Detection

Detection of DVT depends on: clinical suspicion (although clinical diagnosis of a warm, swollen, tender calf is notoriously unreliable), bilateral ascending venography and Doppler ultrasound scanning. Pulmonary embolism may be revealed by a ventilation/perfusion scan. Chest radiographs and an ECG are likely to be more useful for excluding other causes of chest symptoms than in the diagnosis of pulmonary embolism.

Treatment

- For calf vein thrombosis alone: graduated compression stockings and mobilize (low risk of embolism)
- If iliofemoral segment involved: bed rest and anticoagulation with heparin for 7–10 days, then oral warfarin for 3–6 months
- If high risk of embolism, particularly if non-occlusive: thrombolytic therapy or thrombectomy
- For recurrent embolism not controlled by other means, consider insertion of a vena caval filter.

SURGICAL TUBES/DRAINS

In surgical finals, it is useful to decide what a tube attached to the patient may be there for – this may give you helpful information for working out the diagnosis and treatment.

Tubes attached to patients can be either entry tubes (allow something into the body) or exit tubes (let things leave). They can be categorized by function:

- vascular access
  - intravenous line
  - central venous line (fluids/feed/chemotherapy)
  - arterial line (sampling blood/measuring pressures)
  - AV fistula (for dialysis)
- respiratory access
  - endotracheal tube
  - tracheostomy
- gastrointestinal access
  - nasogastric tube (free drainage, continuous/intermittent suction)
  - nasoduodenal tube (feeding)
  - gastrostomy tube (feeding/drainage)
  - jejunostomy tube (feeding)
  - biliary drainage tube (e.g. T tube)

- body cavity access
  - chest drain
  - abdominal drain (suction/free drainage/dialysis tube).

What comes out of the drain can give you a hint as to where the tube is. Nasogastric aspirates may be: opalescent, likened to ginger beer (pure gastric); golden (bile-stained); green (from the small bowel); or faeculent (brown, foul-smelling, from the lower small bowel). Abdominal drains may produce blood, serous fluid, bile or bowel content.

WOUND HEALING

The healing of soft tissue wounds takes 4–5 days on the face and 10–14 days on the trunk and limbs to gain sufficient strength to enable removal of the sutures without disruption to the wound. Further strengthening occurs over about 6 months.

Healing can be by first intention (close and accurate apposition of incised wounds); second intention (defect fills in with granulation tissue and scar contraction shrinks wound size); or third intention (a wound healing by secondary intention is surgically sutured to achieve apposition). Hypertrophic scars (exaggerated normal healing) are raised, red and firm, and may resolve over time. In contrast, keloid scars continue to worsen and enlarge after 6 months.

Factors (particularly adverse factors) affecting wound healing can be divided into general factors and local factors, either of which may occur after any operation or specific to a particular operation.

General factors	Local factors
• age	• site
• jaundice	• tissue damage
• anaemia	• ischaemia
• hypoxia	• bacterial contamination
• steroids	• infection
• immunosuppression	• radiotherapy
• diabetes	• foreign material
• malnutrition	• failure of apposition

For example, wound healing might fail in an elderly diabetic patient (general factors) with a pretibial laceration (site, tissue damage, ischaemia).

WOUND INFECTION

Wounds can be classed as clean (wound contamination not expected, infection rate <1%, e.g. thyroidectomy); clean-contaminated (no frank infection but significant risk of infection, although should be <5%, e.g. cholecystectomy); or contaminated (dirty operations, e.g. surgery for perforated colon).

Prevention of infection should include preoperative skin cleaning (patient's skin and surgeon's hands); reduction in potential contamination (e.g. clearing the colon of faeces before a sigmoid resection); antibiotic prophylaxis against likely contaminating organisms (which may depend on the site, e.g. different for hip replacement and for colonic surgery); and use of sterile equipment.

Signs of wound infection (at 3–4 days postoperatively) include the features of inflammation (hot, red, swollen, tender, loss of function), discharge from the wound, pyrexia and leucocytosis, and (with severe infection) bacteraemia, septicaemia and even death. In contrast, wound haematomata occur earlier (usually with few systemic signs, though they may predispose to infection), and deep wound dehiscence occurs later (at 7–10 days, usually accompanied by a profuse serous discharge followed by the abdominal organs emerging through the wound). However, wound infection may become apparent some time (even years) after surgery, for example related to a nonabsorbable abdominal suture or an orthopaedic prosthesis.

13

Radiology

You may well be asked to look at and comment on a radiograph, as part of a long or a short case or in a viva. You will not be expected to be an expert radiologist but you will be expected to approach a radiograph sensibly, demonstrate a methodical approach to interpreting the films, and detect abnormalities. What are being tested are your approach and your powers of observation. You may be given a short history before you are asked to look at a radiograph, or you may be shown a film from your long or short case. The term 'X-ray' may be used in everyday speech, but is considered bad slang in exams.

There are guidelines which make the interpretation of radiographs (of whatever type) easier, especially in the heat of an exam when all knowledge and reason seem to desert you:

1. Always view the film or films on a well-lit viewing box.
2. Check that the film is the right way up, and orientated correctly with the 'R' marker on what would be the patient's right-hand side if you were standing talking to him or her. If there are several films (e.g. a barium enema series), the examiner will usually choose one for you.
3. Check the patient's name, and date of birth if it is visible.
4. Avoid touching the radiograph thereafter (lots of sweaty fingers during an exam start to irritate the examiners, as the fingers often mark the films). Ask if you want to touch the film.
5. Decide what type of film you are examining: for example, state to the examiner, 'This is an erect chest radiograph of a man.' This makes you sound confident, avoids embarrassing silences, and gives you time to think!
6. Stand back and get an overall impression. Is there a gross abnormality that strikes you immediately?

7. Now study the radiograph systematically: keep talking, stating what you are looking for even if there is no abnormality present – for example, state, 'There is no free air under the diaphragm.'
8. As you spot abnormalities, describe them.
9. Look for a second abnormality, or even more than two.
10. Take a further look to ensure you haven't missed anything that now seems obvious.
11. Summarize what you see. For example, 'This is a double-contrast enema of the colon of a 78-year-old man. There is a mucosal abnormality, with an apple-core deformity in the mid-transverse colon that has the appearance of a colonic carcinoma. There are also radioopaque 1–2 cm lesions on the films, in keeping with calcified mesenteric lymph nodes.'

The aim of this approach to radiographs is to give you a routine. This allows you to demonstrate a systematic way of examining the film, so that you can not only describe the obvious but (with luck) pick up more subtle features which you might otherwise miss. The best way to establish this routine is to practise with a fellow student, a tutor or (preferably) a radiologist, not once but many times, using different films showing different abnormalities. The following examples are intended to complement the radiographs in the companion volume, *Final MB*.

APPROACH TO THE SKULL

1. Always view the film or films on a well-lit viewing box.
2. Check the patient's name, and date of birth if it is visible.
3. Decide what type of film you are examining: a set of skull views of one patient comprises a lateral film, a frontal view and a Towne's view, which focuses on the occiput.
4. Stand back and get an overall impression. Is there a gross abnormality that strikes you immediately?
5. Now study the radiograph systematically, looking at the bony structures then the soft tissues.
6. As you spot abnormalities, describe them.
7. Look for a second abnormality, or even more than two.
8. Take a further look to ensure you haven't missed anything that now seems obvious.
9. Summarize your findings.

Head injury guidelines

You may be asked about the advice you would give to a patient with a minor head injury. Written advice should be given to a relative or friend of any patient who has suffered even a minor head injury. The patient should not:

- be left alone
- be allowed to drive a vehicle or ride a bicycle
- drink alcohol.

After a head injury, a patient who develops any of the following symptoms must be seen by a GP or taken to a hospital as soon as possible:

- confusion or irritability
- drowsiness or difficult to rouse
- severe or progressive headache
- blurred or double vision
- vomiting
- dizziness
- any form of muscle weakness
- slurring or loss of speech
- a fit or seizure.

Case 1

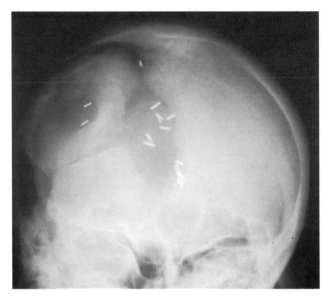

(Answer on page 240)

Case 2

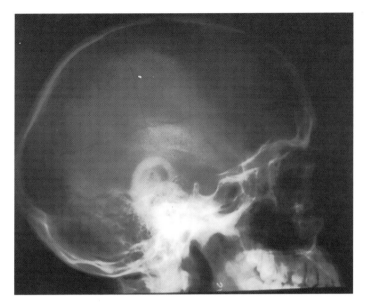

(Answer on page 240)

Case 3

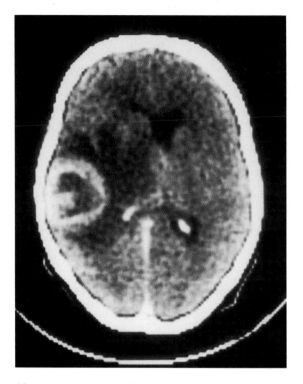

(Answer on page 241)

APPROACH TO THE SPINE

Spinal views are uncommon radiographs for surgical finals, but if used will usually show an obvious abnormality.

1. Always view the film or films on a well-lit viewing box.
2. Check the patient's name, and date of birth if it is visible.
3. Decide what type of film you are examining:
   - views of C1/C2
   - lateral cervical spine/anteroposterior cervical spine view (which should include C7)
   - thoracic spine – lateral/anteroposterior view
   - lumbar/sacral spine – lateral/anteroposterior view.
4. Stand back and get an overall impression. Is there a gross abnormality that strikes you immediately? Are any man-made objects (including jewellery) visible?
5. Now study the radiograph systematically, looking at the bony structures then the soft tissues.
   - For an anteroposterior view, assess the bony structures for:
     - alignment (is any bone obviously out of line with one above or below?)
     - symmetry of the pedicles
     - contour of the vertebral bodies
     - any evidence of bone destruction
     - height of the disc spaces
     - central position of the spinous processes.
   - For a lateral view, assess the bony structures for:
     - alignment of the vertebral bodies/angulation of the spine
     - contour of the vertebral bodies
     - presence of disc spaces
     - width of the spinal canal
   - For a lateral view, assess the soft tissues (especially in the cervical spine) for:
     - widening of the prevertebral space
     - widening of the space between the spinous processes
     - obliteration of the prevertebral (lucent) fat strip.
6. As you spot abnormalities, describe them.
7. Summarize your findings.

Case 4

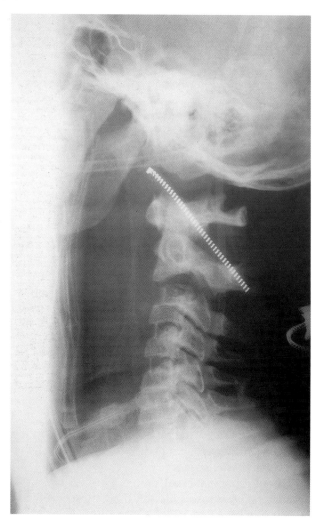

(Answer on page 241)

Case 5

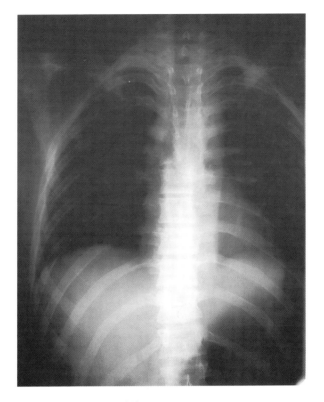

(Answer on page 242)

APPROACH TO THE CHEST

Although a chest radiograph is the film to have for medical finals, it can appear in surgical finals too and may show medical conditions, surgical conditions or both!

1. Always view the film(s) on a well-lit viewing box, and check that the radiograph is correctly orientated.
2. Check the patient's name, and date of birth if it is visible.
3. Decide whether the chest X-ray (oops, remember not to use that X-rated term!) is a posteroanterior (PA) or anteroposterior (AP) view, and whether the film was taken with the patient erect. A PA view is the standard view, though an AP view (on which the letters 'AP' should be written) may be taken outwith the Radiology Department. So what? Does this matter? Yes: in a PA view, the cardiothoracic ratio (ratio of transverse size of cardiac outline to transverse size of the thoracic cage) is normally less than 0.5. In an AP view, the heart is effectively magnified and so you should not comment on cardiomegaly. An erect chest film (PA view) is used as the standard way to detect intraperitoneal gas, as 'free gas under the diaphragm'.
4. Is there a gross abnormality?
5. Systematically talk your way through the film:
   * heart and mediastinal structures
   * lung fields
   * pleurae, diaphragm and below the diaphragm
   * bony structures
     - humerei
     - scapulae
     - clavicles
     - cervical/thoracic spine
     - ribs
   * soft tissues
     - breasts (has there been a mastectomy?)
     - subcutaneous tissues (chest/neck/arms; is there any surgical emphysema?)
6. Take a final look and draw your thoughts together.
7. Summarize what you can see.

Case 6

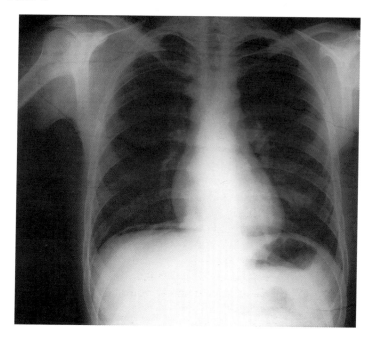

(Answer on page 242)

Case 7

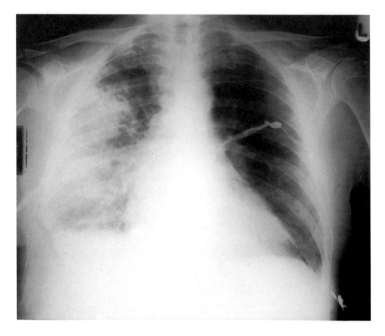

(Answer on page 243)

Case 8a

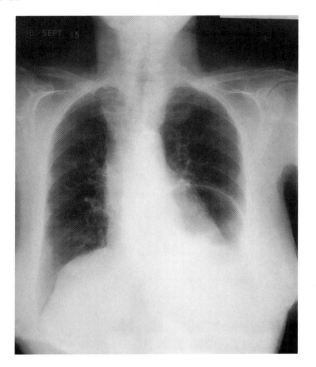

Case 8b

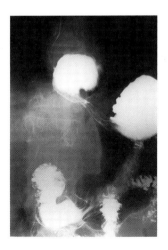

(Answer on page 244)

Case 9

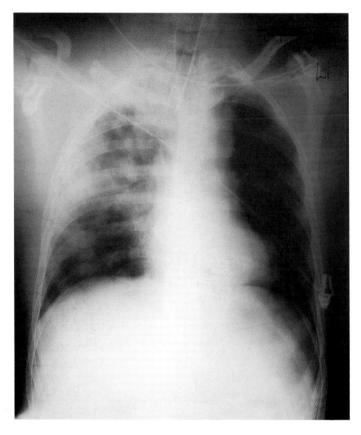

(Answer on page 245)

Case 10

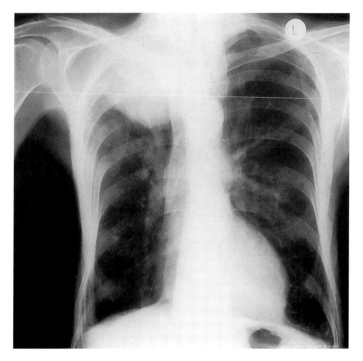

(Answer on page 245)

Case 11

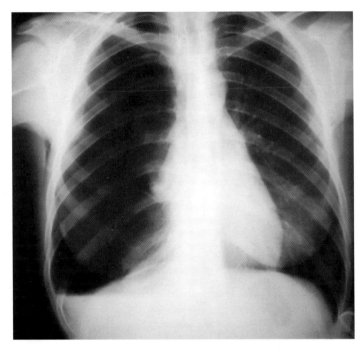

(Answer on page 246)

Case 12

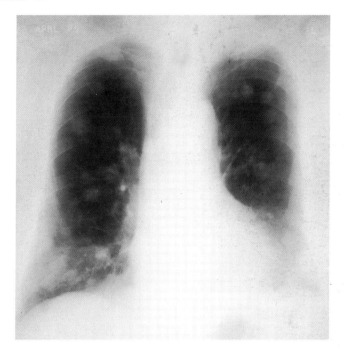

(Answer on page 246)

Case 13

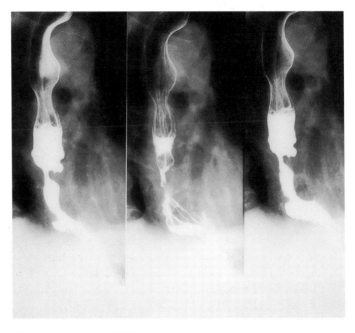

(Answer on page 247)

APPROACH TO THE BREAST

Breast screening for malignancy, by mammography, is in common usage in many countries. Mammograms detect abnormal densities, calcification, parenchymal deformities and spiculate masses in contrast to the surrounding breast tissue. Because of the density of the breast tissue of young women, mammography is usually confined to women over 35 years of age. In national breast screening programmes, mammography is performed on women of 50–64 years of age (or from age 40 years to 70 years in some programmes), every 18 months-3 years.

1. Always view the mammogram film or films on a well-lit viewing box, and ask for a magnifying glass (to look particularly for microcalcification).
2. Check the patient's name, and date of birth if it is visible.
3. Decide what type of film you are examining: the film should be marked 'L' or 'R' to indicate which breast it shows. For each side, there should be a craniocaudal view (marked 'CC' on the film) and an oblique view (marked 'OBL').
4. Stand back and get an overall impression. Is there a gross abnormality that strikes you immediately? There usually will be: an obvious cancer may stand out as a spiculate mass like 'a star in the night'.
5. Now study each mammogram systematically, looking at the breast tissue for opacities (size, shape, contour, number), asymmetry and parenchymal deformity.
6. As you spot abnormalities, describe them.
7. Look for a second abnormality, or even more than two, on each side.
8. Check for abnormally dense lymph nodes in the axilla.
9. Take a further look to ensure you haven't missed anything that now seems obvious.
10. Summarize what you can see.

Case 14

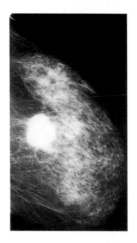

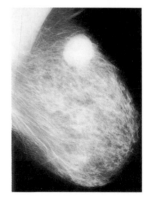

(Answer on page 247)

APPROACH TO THE ABDOMEN

Abdominal radiographs of one sort or another are the most frequently encountered films in surgical finals. Like chest radiographs, they often have more than one abnormality and respond well to the thought, 'Don't panic, I *can* work through this radiograph systematically, and detect the abnormalities.'

1. Check that the film is correctly orientated and on a well-lit viewing box.
2. Check the patient's name, and date of birth if it is visible.
3. Decide what sort of film you are examining. Is it a plain radiograph, or has contrast been introduced into the patient? If there is contrast, is it inside the bowel (upper gastrointestinal tract, small bowel, colon) or inside another structure (biliary tree, vascular tree)? For gastrointestinal tract contrast examinations, is this a single-contrast study (i.e. a contrast agent such as barium) or a double-contrast study (e.g. barium + air, to give enhanced mucosal detail)? A computed tomography (CT) or magnetic resonance imaging (MRI) scan series can find its way to exams. The examiner should ask you to look at one or two sections in particular. At first, CT scans and MRI scans can be really intimidating, but go through the same systematic process and you will at least detect the main abnormality.
4. Is there a gross abnormality?
5. Proceed to describe the film systematically:
   - hollow viscera (stomach/intestines; bowel gas pattern)
   - solid viscera (kidneys/liver outline; gas in the biliary tree)
   - vascular structures (calcification in the wall)
   - bony structures
     - pelvic bones (contour and consistency)
     - thoracic/lumbar/sacral spine
     - ribs
     - femoral heads
   - subcutaneous tissues (lower chest, abdomen, pelvis).
6. Take a final look and draw your thoughts together.
7. Summarize what you can see.

Case 15a

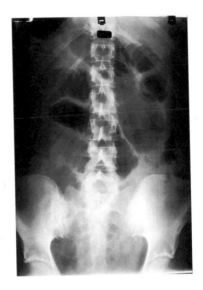

Case 15b

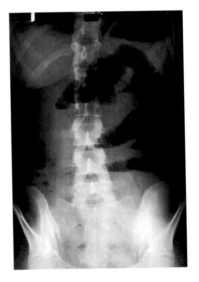

(Answer on page 248)

Case 16

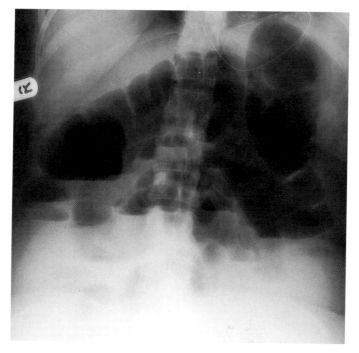

(Answer on page 248)

Case 17

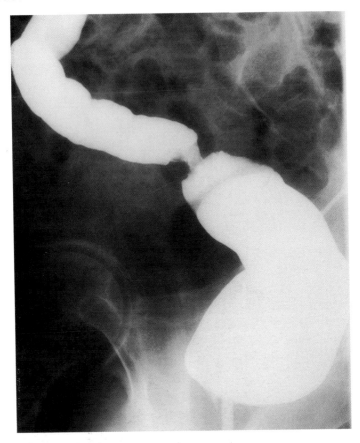

(Answer on page 249)

Case 18

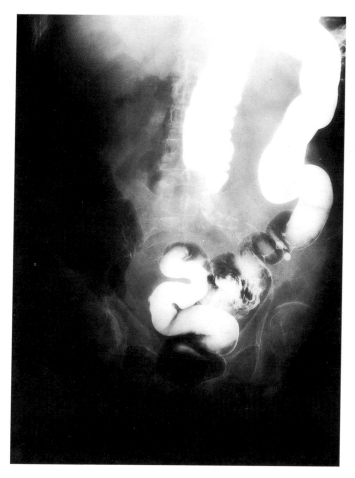

(Answer on page 249)

Case 19

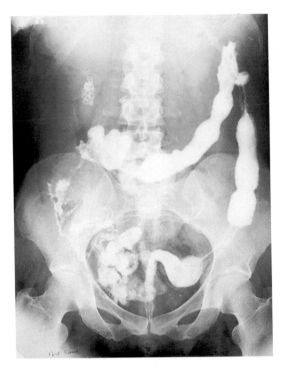

(Answer on page 250)

Case 20

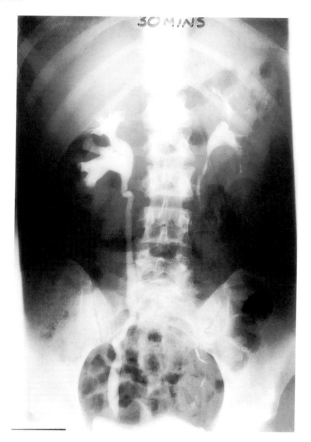

(Answer on page 250)

Case 21

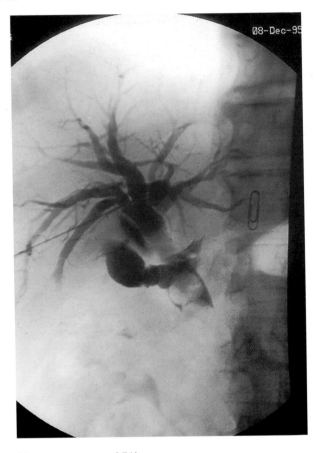

08-Dec-95

(Answer on page 251)

Case 22

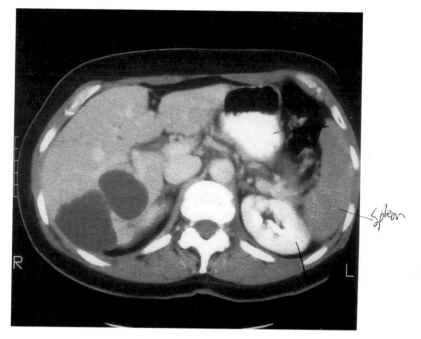

(Answer on page 251)

Case 23

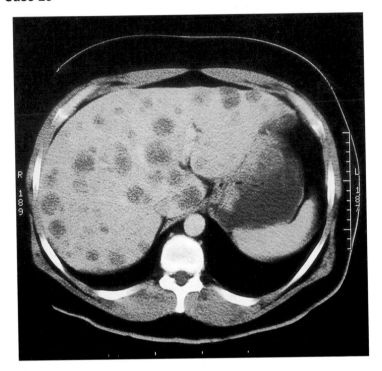

(Answer on page 252)

APPROACH TO THE LIMBS

1. Always view the film or films on a well-lit viewing box.
2. Check the patient's name, and date of birth if it is visible.
3. Decide what type of film you are examining: is it a plain radiograph or is there contrast (e.g. an angiogram)? Plain radiographs aimed at detecting bone or joint abnormalities should include two views of the bone or joint in question and, for bones, the joints proximal and distal to the bone under study.
4. Stand back and get an overall impression. Is there a gross abnormality that strikes you immediately?
5. Now study the radiograph systematically, looking at:
   - bony structures:
     - is there an obvious bone deformity?
     - are the contours of the bones smooth and unbroken in outline?
     - are there prostheses present?
   - soft tissues:
     - is there a joint effusion (fat pad sign)?
     - is there contrast in the vascular tree (an angiogram)?
     - is there vascular calcification?
     - is there subcutaneous swelling?
     - is there gas in the tissue planes?
6. As you spot abnormalities, describe them.
7. Look for a second abnormality, or even more than two.
8. Take a further look to ensure you haven't missed anything that now seems obvious.
9. Summarize your findings.

Case 24

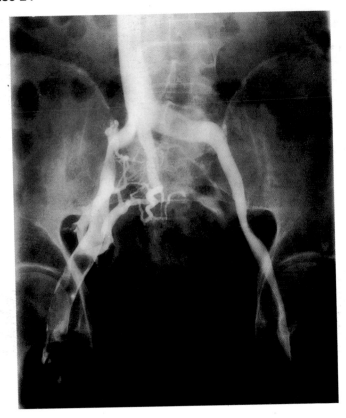

(Answer on page 252)

Case 25

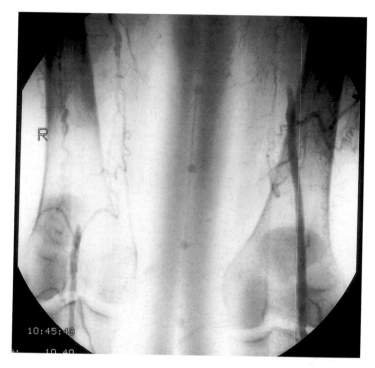

(Answer on page 253)

Case 26

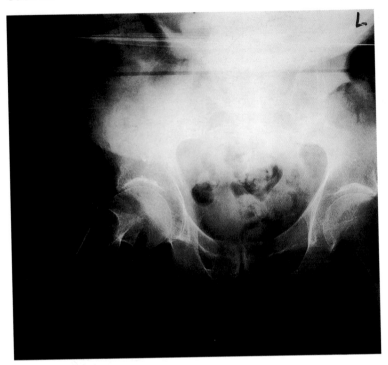

(Answer on page 253)

Case 27

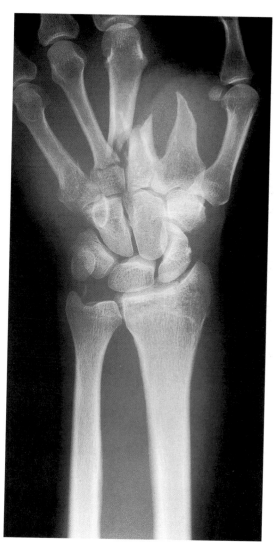

(Answer on page 254)

Case 28

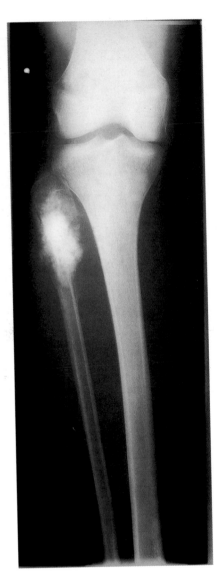

(Answer on page 254)

Case 29

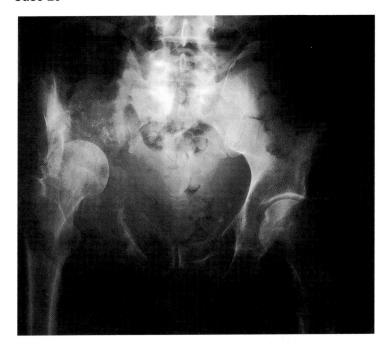

(Answer on page 255)

Case 30a

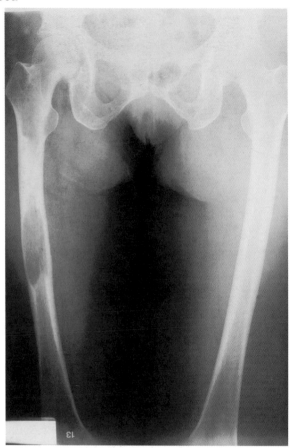

Case 30b

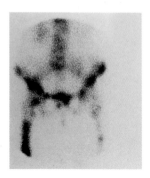

(Answer on page 255)

Case 31

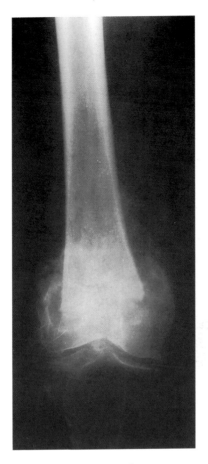

(Answer on page 256)

Case 1

Findings

- This is a frontal skull radiograph.
- There are four bony discontinuities in the vault of the skull on one side.
- There are several metal surgical clips.
- There is no obvious soft tissue swelling.

Summary

There has been severe bony injury, and subsequent surgery to one side of the skull.
   (Cause: machine gun round.)

Case 2

Findings

- This is a lateral skull radiograph.
- There is a fracture line passing transversely from the frontal bone, across the temporal and parietal bones, as far as the lambdoid suture.

Summary

There is a linear fracture of the skull.
   (Cause: blow to the head.)

Case 3

Findings

- This is a CT scan of the head.
- There is a single space occupying lesion in the left cerebral cortex.
- The lesion is associated with occlusion of the left ventricle and midline shift to the right.

Summary

Space occupying lesion in the left cerebral cortex, causing mid line shift.

(Cause: single secondary brain metastasis from breast cancer primary.)

Case 4

Findings

- This is a lateral cervical spine radiograph of C1–C7.
- There is misalignment of C2/C3 and C3/C4.
- There is a crush fracture of C3.
- There is increased space between C2 and C3.
- There are two metallic objects (parts of a zip?) on the radiograph, and two barely radioopaque tubes passing across the field of view.

Summary

There is a major cervical injury, with fracture dislocation of C3.

(This radiograph emphasizes the importance of the 'A' (airway with cervical spine control) in the ABC of resuscitation.)

Case 5

Findings

- This is a posteroanterior (PA) view of the chest.
- There is gross misalignment of the thoracic spine at T6.
- There is a fracture through the body of the sixth thoracic vertebra.
- There are no apparent rib fractures or obvious soft tissue injuries.

Summary

Displaced fracture of the sixth thoracic spine.
   (Cause: fall from ladder.)

Case 6

Findings

- This is an erect PA chest radiograph of a young male (no breasts; no calcification in the costal cartilages).
- There is free air under the right hemidiaphragm.
- Heart, lung fields, bony structures and soft tissues are otherwise normal.

Summary

Free intraperitoneal air under the right hemidiaphragm in a young man.
   (Cause: a perforated duodenal ulcer.)

Case 7

Findings

- This is a chest radiograph.
- There is opacification of the right lung field, worst in the lower and mid-zones.
- There is blunting of the right costophrenic angle.
- There appear to be two ECG leads attached to the patient's chest.

There are no obvious abnormalities of the bony structures or other soft tissues.

Summary

Opacification of the lower three-quarters of the right lung field, and a small pleural effusion.

(Cause: aspiration pneumonia, secondary to an obstructing oesophageal cancer.)

Case 8a

Findings

- This is a PA chest radiograph of a woman.
- There is a gas-filled viscus, with gas/fluid levels, in the left lower lung field.
- The left cardiac border is unusually straight.
- There are no other obvious abnormalities in the lung fields (including no evidence of aspiration), or of the bony structures or soft tissues.

Summary

There is a large gas/fluid filled viscus in the lower left thorax.
    (Cause: in this patient, there was a large rolling hiatus hernia, which had become ischaemic and symptomatic.)

Case 8b

Findings

- This radiograph was taken after introducing a contrast meal.
- There is contrast outlining the oesophagus, stomach, duodenum and jejunum.
- There is a hiatus hernia outlined by contrast above the diaphragm.

Summary

A moderately large hiatus hernia.

Case 9

Findings

- This is a supine chest radiograph, taken at 9 pm.
- The film shows opacification of the right, upper and middle lung fields, and a fractured right clavicle.
- There is an endotracheal tube in place, and three ECG leads are attached to the patient.

Summary

Supine chest radiograph, showing right, upper and middle lung field opacification and a fractured right clavicle in an intubated, monitored patient.

(Cause: road traffic accident.)

Case 10

Findings

- This is a PA chest radiograph.
- There is a rounded opacity in the right upper lung field.

Summary

Opacity in upper right lung field.

(Cause: bronchogenic carcinoma of the right lung – Pancoast tumour.)

Case 11

Findings

- This is a PA chest radiograph of a woman.
- There is a large right pneumothorax, demonstrated by the absence of vascular markings in the right lung field (compared with the left side).
- There is blunting of the right costophrenic angle.

Summary

Right pneumothorax, with fluid level in the costophrenic angle on the same side.

(Cause: haemopneumothorax following attempted central venous line insertion into right subclavian vein.)

Case 12

Findings

- This is a plain radiograph of the chest.
- There are multiple rounded opacities (coin lesions) throughout both lung fields.
- There is opacification of the base of the left and to a lesser extent right lung fields suggestive of pneumonia.

Summary

There are multiple pulmonary nodules plus bilateral basal bronchopneumonia.

(Cause: metastases from renal clear cell carcinoma with pneumonia secondary to occlusion of bronchi by tumour nodules.)

Case 13

Findings

- These are three lateral views of the chest taken during a double-contrast (air + contrast medium) swallow.
- There is a partially obstructing exophytic lesion in the lower third of the oesophagus.

Summary

This is a double-contrast swallow, demonstrating an exophytic lesion in the lower oesophagus.
   (Cause: carcinoma of the lower oesophagus.)

Case 14

Findings

- These are craniocaudal and oblique mammograms of the same breast, L or R not marked.
- There is an opacity in the upper outer quadrant of the breast, visible on both views.
- Part of the margin of the lesion is indistinct.
- There are no visible axillary lymph nodes.

Summary

There is what is radiologically a breast carcinoma in the upper outer quadrant of the breast.

Case 15

Findings

- These films are plain abdominal radiographs taken with the patient supine (15a) and erect (15b).
- There are multiple distended gas filled loops of small bowel (small bowel as the folds of mucosa pass right across the diameter of the small bowel; colonic haustrations pass only part way across the diameter) (15a).
- There are multiple air/fluid levels in the small bowel and in the stomach (15b).
- There is no air apparent in the colon.

Summary

These radiographs show multiple distended small bowel loops suggesting small bowel obstruction.

(Cause: small bowel obstruction due to an obstructing caecal carcinoma.)

Case 16

Findings

- This is a plain abdominal film. Although it does not state so, it is a film taken with the patient erect.
- A distended transverse colon, hepatic flexure and gas/fluid levels can be seen.
- There are multiple gas/fluid levels in the small bowel.
- There is a nasogastric tube in place.

Summary

The distribution of the gas/fluid levels suggests large bowel obstruction.

(Cause: colonic obstruction due to a descending colonic carcinoma.)

Case 17

Findings

- This radiograph was taken after introducing a single-contrast enema.
- There is an apple-core deformity at the rectosigmoid junction.

Summary

An apple-core lesion of the colon, shown on contrast enema. (Cause: rectosigmoid carcinoma.)

Case 18

Findings

- This radiograph was taken after introducing a contrast enema, most of which is single-contrast, although there is double-contrast (air + radiological contrast) in the sigmoid colon.
- There is a shouldered cut-off to the flow of contrast, and a distended caecum proximally, suggestive of a colon cancer.
- There are also two sigmoid diverticulae.
- The bifurcation of the aorta and common iliac arteries are calcified.
- There is loss of the joint space and osteosclerosis of the right hip, suggesting osteoarthritis.

Summary

There is an obstructing transverse colon lesion and also diverticular disease, vascular calcification and osteoarthritis of the right hip.
   (Cause: obstructing transverse colon carcinoma; incidental diverticular disease, calcified common iliac vessels, and osteoarthritis of the hip.)

Case 19

Findings

- This radiograph was taken after introducing a contrast enema of the colon.
- There are strictures of the transverse and descending colon separated by normal segments of colon.

Summary

Colonic strictures (skip lesions) compatible with Crohn's disease.
   (Cause: Crohn's disease.)

Case 20

Findings

- This is the 30-minute film from an intravenous urogram (IVU) or IVP (intravenous pyelography) series.
- There is dilation of the right ureter and pelvicalyceal system, with a cut-off at the lower end of the ureter.
- There is a functioning left kidney.
- A control film should be reviewed, to look for radioopaque stones.

Summary

This IVU shows a low right ureteric obstruction.
   (Cause: stone at the lower end of the right ureter, subsequently passed spontaneously.)

Case 21

Findings

- This is a percutaneous transhepatic cholangiogram (PTC; note the contrast in the needle, and the absence of an endoscope and surgical implements).
- There are two large common bile duct stones, one obstructing the duct.
- There is biliary tree dilation and filling of the gallbladder.
- There is a paper-clip (a skin marker) visible on the film.

Summary

This PTC shows large gallstones obstructing the common bile duct.

(Cause: large gallstones obstructing the common bile duct; ERCP had been unsuccessful.)

Case 22

Findings

- This is an abdominal computed tomography (CT) scan.
- It is an image taken through the liver.
- The scan shows two lesions in the right lobe of the liver.
- The patient has contrast (barium) in the stomach, and has had intravenous contrast (being excreted via the visible, left, kidney on this view). The spleen is also seen.

Summary

There are two lesions in the right lobe of the liver on this section of an abdominal CT scan.

(Cause: benign liver cysts.)

Case 23

Findings

- This is a CT scan of the abdomen through the liver, stomach and spleen.
- There are multiple lesions throughout the liver indicative of metastases.
- The wall of the stomach adjacent to the liver (the lesser curve) is thickened with a mass protruding into the lumen of the stomach.

Summary

This CT scan of the upper abdomen shows multiple liver metastases and an abnormal stomach.

(Cause: adenocarcinoma of the lesser curve of the stomach with multiple liver metastases.)

Case 24

Findings

- This is a pelvic radiograph, showing intravenous contrast from a bilateral femoral vein puncture.
- The venogram has outlined the ileofemoral veins and vena cava, demonstrating thrombus in the right and left ileo-femoral segments.

Summary

Deep venous thrombosis.

(Cause: postoperative DVT after abdominal surgery; the patient subsequently had a pulmonary embolus.)

Case 25

Findings

- This is one of a series of arteriograms of the lower limbs.
- The femoral artery is occluded on both sides and there appears to be a longer occluded segment on the right, although the proximal extent is not visible from this single film.
- There is good collateral circulation, filling the distal femoral/popliteal arteries.
- Further views should be examined to determine the extent of disease in the lower limbs.

Summary

Bilateral femoral artery occlusions, with collateral circulation.
   (Cause: atherosclerosis.)

Case 26

Findings

- This is an incomplete plain radiograph of the pelvis.
- There is a fracture of the neck of the right femur.

Summary

Fracture of the neck of the femur.
   (Cause: fall at home.)

Case 27

Findings

- This is a plain radiograph of the wrist, carpal and metacarpal bones.
- There is an amputation of the 2nd metacarpal through the shaft; it is an old amputation since new cortical bone has formed over the cut bone surface.
- There is a fracture through the shaft of the 3rd metacarpal.
- There is a fracture of the base of the 4th metacarpal.
- There is a fracture through the joint surface of the head of the radius.

Summary

Old 2nd metacarpal amputation; multiple new fractures of the carpal bones and radial head.

(Cause: previous traumatic amputation; further trauma due to road traffic accident.)

Case 28

Findings

- This is a plain radiograph of the proximal tibia and fibula and distal femur.
- There is a radiodense mass in the proximal fibula, destroying the normal architecture.
- Distal to the tumour, the periosteum appears to be raised.

Summary

Tumour of the proximal fibula.

(Cause: osteosarcoma.)

Case 29

Findings

- This is a plain radiograph of the pelvis.
- There is destruction of all but the iliac crest of the bones of the right hemipelvis.
- There is dislocation of the right femur as a consequence of the pelvic destruction.
- There is faecal loading of the colon and rectum (possibly secondary to the use of analgesics).

Summary

Destruction of the right hemipelvis, with dislocation of the femur.

(Cause: metastatic prostate cancer.)

Case 30

Findings

- This is a plain radiograph of the lower pelvis and shafts of left and right femurs (30a).
- There are lytic areas in the midshaft of the right femur and in the neck of the femur.
- This is a static isotope bone scan showing the lumbar spine, pelvis and upper femurs (30b).
- There are hot spots (dark areas on the film) indicating bone metastases in the right femoral shaft (corresponding to the lytic area on 30a) but also in the pelvis.

Summary

Osteolytic bone metastasis in the right femoral midshaft and pelvis.

(Cause: multiple bone metastases from a primary breast cancer.)

Case 31

Findings

- This is a plain radiograph of the lower femur.
- There is a displaced fracture of the distal femur.
- There is callus formation around the fracture site.
- There is osteopaenia of the tibia and (barely visible) fibula.

Summary

Healing fracture of the distal shaft of the femur.
   (Cause: road traffic accident.)

Index